Transform Mind and Body with the Lap-Band

Awaken to a Life No Longer Controlled by Hunger and Weight

**Lisa Gentile, MS, RD, CPFT-HFI,
Certified Integrative Nutritionist**

ISBN: 1456528009
ISBN-13: 9781456528003

Table of Contents

Acknowledgements

I am grateful for all the physicians who have devoted their lives to helping those who suffer from obesity. I would especially like to thank Dr. Richard Rubenstein whose pioneering dedication into bariatric medicine initially encouraged me to devote my efforts toward helping those who struggle with this deadly disease. My gratitude is extended to Dr. Alan Geiss, and the entire Bariatric programs offered at North Shore Long Island Jewish for giving me the opportunity to practice at the highest level of bariatric care.

Personally, to my mother and father whose perseverance in the face of their terminal illness inspired me to pursue my deepest interests. In addition, I would like to acknowledge Theresa, who in spite of unsuccessful bariatric surgeries, she continues her arduous journey towards attaining a healthier body weight.

To my boy Joshua, your beautiful captivating artwork was a perfect inspiration to this project. I know this is just the beginning of displaying your inner most creativity. To my daughter Olivia, you exemplify the meaning of Liv-(ing) – I love you both dearly.

Lastly, to the thousands of patients I have had the utmost privilege in consulting and working with. Your expertise in living with the Lap-Band has allowed me to be a vessel of knowledge to others in need.

A Brief Overview of Obesity

Obesity is defined as a disease in which excess fat accumulates to the extent that it may adversely affect health.[1] The prevalence of obesity has dramatically increased within the U.S. population over the past few decades. Statistics have shown that this chronic progressive disease, which reflects the convergence of many biological, economic, and social factors, has reached alarming proportions.[2] It is currently estimated that 26.4 million Americans are obese with approximately 8.4 million suffering from morbid obesity.[3]

With conservative management of obesity, consisting of nutrition, pharmacological therapy, behavior modification, and exercise displaying a 90 percent failure rate,[4] physicians have worked endlessly to develop a truly effective modality of treatment. Their efforts have led to the development of a number of effective surgical techniques designed to reduce food consumption and/or absorption in order to facilitate permanent weight loss. Recent statistics have reported that two hundred thousand surgeries were performed in 2010 for the treatment of obesity with approximately fifty percent performed of the Lap-Band.[5]

Back in 1990, The National Institute of Health (NIH) concluded that "diets, exercise, behavioral modification, and even pharmacological drugs almost always fail in the obese population".[6] Furthermore, The National Heart, Lung and Blood Institute's Expert Panel on Identification, Evaluation and Treatment of Overweight and Obesity has recognized "obesity surgery as the only long-term, effective treatment for morbid obesity".[7] Despite positive legislation, weight loss surgeries are still considered predominantly "elective". This premise still exists because of the fact that these procedures are not considered "absolutely" medically necessary; however, those individuals who suffer from the storage of excess body weight know quite differently. The suffering of million Americans has led the crusade of bariatric (obesity) surgical treatment.

As bariatric medicine has expanded, so have the qualifications distinguishing those individuals who are most suitable for surgical intervention. Aside from gender, genetics, weight history, previous attempts to manage weight, and medical history; criteria for surgical candidacy is still primarily rooted in the body mass index, BMI.

The body mass index is a calculation intended to standardize an individual's body weight in comparison to their height. The specific formula to determine BMI is as follows: (weight in kilograms) divided by (height in meters squared).

The first step in attaining a BMI is to determine weight in kilograms through dividing a given weight in pounds by 2.2. The second step involves converting height into meters (squared) through multiplying height in inches by .254, (squared).

As an example, a person weighing 150 pounds at 5 feet, 5 inches tall would calculate their BMI as follows: Divide 150 by 2.2 = 68 kilograms; multiply 65 inches (5 feet, 5 inches in height) by .254 = 16.5 height in meters. Next, square 16.5 by multiplying 16.5 x 16.5 = 272. Final step: divide 68 kilograms by 272 for a BMI of 25.

Categorically, a BMI between 18.5 and 24.9 is normal whereas a value from 25.0 to 29.9 is considered overweight. Obesity is then graded as mild - Class I (30.0 to 34.9 BMI), moderate - Class II (35.0 to 39.9 BMI), and morbid - Class III (40.0 + BMI).[8]

Due to the unwavering association between morbid obesity and a vast array of medical conditions (co-morbidities) that present with serious risk of mortality (including high blood pressure, diabetes, high cholesterol, cardiovascular disease, degenerative joint disease, and pulmonary dysfunction, along with social and psychiatric abnormalities), insurance companies have traditionally covered the cost of obesity surgery for those candidates who present with a BMI of 40 and greater, or a BMI between 35-39 with one or more co-morbidities. Recently, the U.S. Food and Drug Administration (FDA) approved the Lap-Band system for adults with a BMI of 30-35 and who are also suffering with at least one related co-morbid condition.[9]

Statistics reveal that the incidence of morbid obesity has increased at double the rate of obesity, which is reflected in the increasing yearly rate of weight loss surgeries. The World Health Organization characterized the relative rise in morbid obesity (over the exponential rise in obesity) as an "epidemic within an epidemic."[10] Together, the medical conditions associated with morbid obesity have accounted for nearly two-thirds of the deaths occurring each year in the United States.[11] Worldwide, documentation shows that greater than 2.5 million deaths per year are in fact weight-related.[12]

1.   Buchwald, H., 2005.
2.   Alfred, J.B., 1995.
3.   Allergan Lap-Band system, 2011
4.   Buchwald, H., 2002.
5.   Allergan Lap-Band system, 2011
6.   Buffington, C., 2004.
7.   Craig, M.R. et al., 2000.
8.   Martin, L.F., 2004.
9.   Allergen Lap-Band System, 2011
10.   United Health Organization, 2000.
11.   Craig, M.R. et al., 2000.
12.   Deitel, M., 2003.

Bariatric Surgical Weight Loss Treatment

Medical science has designated the term "bariatrics" to represent the specialized treatment of obesity. The respective operations are thus regarded as bariatric surgeries. The main effects of bariatric surgery are to enhance fullness (satiation) and reduce subjective hunger.[1]

Three categories of bariatric operations are presently recognized:

1. restrictive, which reduce food consumption and thus caloric intake;
2. malabsorptive, which reduce total caloric uptake/absorption by the body; and
3. operations that possess a combination of both malabsorption and restriction.

Prior to FDA-approval in 2001 for the first laparoscopic adjustable gastric banding (LAGB) specifically, the Lap-Band System (Inamed Health, Santa Barbara, CA), stomach stapling was the only surgical option.[2] Although gastric banding is relatively new in the US, with approximately ten years experience in the general population, Europe and Australia have been using gastric bands since the early 1980s. Even so, gastric bypass surgery continues to be a common weight loss surgery performed in the United States. Gastric bypass surgery became increasingly popular because this procedure offers both restriction of intake along with an anatomical component that reduces the absorption of calories.

Although gastric bypass is still considered a "golden standard" of bariatric surgery, LAGB has become more widely accepted during the past several years. Researchers believe LAGB will soon overshadow bypass surgery because it entails a minimally invasive surgical technique that does not alter the anatomy with a highly comparable long-term success rate. Continuation in normal digestive processes ensures full nutrient absorption, thus eliminating the risk of nutritional and/or vitamin deficiencies that are quite possible among more invasive type surgeries, like gastric bypass. In addition, the LAGB procedure is both reversible and adjustable. Reversibility in that the band can be removed while leaving the anatomy in normal structure. Adjustability of the opening to the lower stomach thereby influencing the degree of physical intake restriction.

1. Dixon, J.B., 2005.
2. Favretti, F. et al., 1993.

The Uniqueness of the Lap-Band

Designation of the "Lap-Band" System is quite simple to visualize—the term *Lap* refers to the only surgical technique utilized to implant this physical apparatus, laparoscopic. Secondly, the belt-like, rubber band configuration of the apparatus is representative of the terminology *Band*. The Lap-Band (band) is a purely restrictive procedure, which is designed to reduce food intake by imposing external constriction of the stomach. The procedure divides the stomach into two parts. The area above the band is commonly referred to as the "pouch" whereas the area below the band represents the remaining lower area of the stomach.

The restrictive element of the operation involves creating a small "virtual" pouch at the top portion of the stomach. This pouch possesses a miniature outlet (made possible by the placement of the band) to the lower (larger) stomach area. Configuration of the pouch not only promotes reduction of intake, but also upon distention of food consumption, comfortable satiation is achieved shortly after the meal begins. The restrictive, slow movement of food flowing through the pouch to the lower stomach and eventually continuing on the digestive path also promotes satiation long after a meal is completed.

Although placement of the band is a simple process involving a straightforward mechanical technique, it does possess a dynamic effect. This dynamic effect allows recipients of this tool to be alleviated from abnormal fluctuations in *hunger*—the physiological sensation that drives the ingestion of calories. Placement of the band at the junction of the esophagus and stomach is believed to help stimulate nerves that reside in an area of the brain called the hypothalamus. The hypothalamus provides a feedback mechanism for subtlety suppressing the physiological desire for food. In essence, Lap-Band surgery allows for the attainment of profound *satiety*—a physiological sensation that inhibits the ingestion of food and subsequently fewer calories.

Piecing the factors together helps visualize the innate characteristics of the Lap-Band device as a means of (1) decreasing hunger, (2) curtailing eating, and (3) enhancing cognitive-thoughtful restraint.

The absence of extreme physical hunger, which too often plagues weight-challenged individuals, helps to inhibit eating all together. Curtailing the desire for food has been shown to enhance the preponderance for well-balanced, nourishing foods while promoting greater cognitive restraint. With this in mind, it is noteworthy to understand that restraint from eating high calorie, slippery foods (foods that 'slide' through the opening because of inadequate texture) while living with the band will promote superior weight loss. Slippery, high calorie foods including ice cream, cookies, and cake are much easier to consume after surgery because these snacks lack solid consistency and as a result, fail to produce optimal satiation. Optimal satiation is obtained through the intake of high quality foods such as lean protein and vegetables both of solid to semi-solid consistency. Solid to semi-solid consistency protein and vegetable-based foods provide bulky-dense textures, which remain in the upper pouch for the longest length of time.

After recognizing adequate satiation, post-banded patients can once again learn to eat based on innate feelings of their appetite. They no longer struggle with eating past the point of feeling full because of inadequate satiety. It is up to the individual however to determine when, how much, and the most suitable "meal mix"—a balance of protein, carbohydrate, and fat that will best meet their physiological needs.

Unlike other surgical procedures that create a restrictive pouch through suturing the stomach, the Lap-Band's internal circumference can be modified in an effort to meet the needs of each individual patient. During the post-operative phase, a skilled practitioner can adjust the opening between the upper stomach pouch and the remaining lower stomach by inflating saline into the lining of the silicone band. Saline solution is dispensed by means of a thin needle onto the surface of the skin directed through a port. The port is connected to the band by way of tubing and is implanted beneath the abdominal cavity at the time of surgery. Patients describe a light pinch of the skin while saline is delivered through the port.

The balloon encompassing the band can be restricted or unrestricted through administering or releasing saline. Inflating the band with saline increases distention in the upper stomach pouch and stomach, thus producing a quick and profound feeling of comfortable fullness when eating. If necessary, the opening can also be modified by aspirating fluid from the band. Leaving the band with less saline creates a larger opening from the upper stomach pouch to the remaining lower stomach region. This may be necessary to provide for adequate intake and/or optimal tolerance if in fact key habits are not well established. These essential eating habits include chewing food thoroughly before swallowing and eating at a very slow pace, while simultaneously devoting fully focused attention to the meal at hand. Performing all of these necessary habits will also require eating within a non-distracted, relaxing environment.

Adjusting the Lap-Band

Adjustments, or what are commonly referred to as "fills," are performed in the post-operative phase once tissue-swelling (edema) surrounding the band subsides. Swelling inevitably occurs as result of placing the band. The extent and length of time for swelling to exist varies with each individual, however it generally occurs for several weeks after surgery. Due to unpredictable tissue swelling, it has been common practice to leave the band empty or "unfilled" at the time of surgery. If the band is filled at the time of surgery (as some surgeons have recently started to experiment with), the intake of full liquids may in fact be very challenging, as the opening between the pouch and the lower stomach presents extremely occluded from the swelling. Nutritional adequacy could then be of notable concern.

Placing a band that is without a fill will also ensure that the internal surgical area has time to heal adequately without the possibility of having trouble with intake. These difficulties can include pain when drinking too quickly, or even more problematic, slippage of the band. The risk of slipping the band during the initial healing period is significantly increased with the occurrence of regurgitation or vomiting. The forceful movement accompanied by regurgitation or vomiting places unnecessary stress on the newly placed band. This stress can make the band more prone to slip from the original surgical position while trying to form an adhesive closure with the surrounding stomach tissue. If the band should slip (or prolapse as referred to in the bariatric medical field) at any point in time, repositioning can be done by simply removing saline so the band can reconfigure to the original position. If this is unsuccessful, then surgery may be required to realign the band to the stomach.

Keep in mind that changing a patient's lifelong habits surrounding his/her relationship with food (including eating at an extremely slow pace while adequately chewing food) can be overwhelming and may require extensive practice. Taking time after surgery to establish these habits before additional restriction is placed on the food passageway is both a safe and smart decision.

In addition to these premises, 5 to 10 percent of Lap-Band recipients will never require an adjustment because the restriction provided by an unfilled band is more than sufficient to limit intake while triggering adequate satiety stimulation. For the remaining 90 to 95 percent of Lap-Band recipients who will eventually require adjustments, it is considered best to wait until…

1. a solid food plan is consumed with adequate tolerance and
2. an indication for an adjustment is recognized by means of
    a. insufficient weight loss or
    b. ineffective satiation at and between meals.

The majority of bariatric programs recommend waiting until the patient has successfully adapted to the intake of solid foods for at least two weeks before considering an adjustment. If a patient should, however, indicate a definite need for an adjustment as determined by weight loss goals (e.g., weight loss has not advanced favorably) as well as an array of pertinent dietary factors (e.g., capacity to consume is much greater then recommended), then this intervention can be handled individually with his or her physician. Indication that an initial adjustment is needed sooner than anticipated signifies that there may not have been prominent swelling encompassing the band upon surgical placement.

Consuming solid foods on a regular basis is one of the highest priorities after surgery. Solid foods are most suitable to consume because initial and prolonged satiation can be achieved more effectively when foods are of dense texture. It is of prime importance to ensure optimal tolerance of these foods before restrictive modification within the diameter of the band is granted.

In addition to these considerations, there are individual factors that must be reviewed when making the decision to have or not have an adjustment. These factors include:

(A). Insufficient weight loss
(B). Lack of satiation during a meal along with inadequate satiety between meals

(A)   Insufficient weight loss

Although losing less weight than anticipated is a true concern from some, it is important to consider individual aspects that govern metabolism and the catabolic effect of fat breakdown. Considering these aspects will provide for accurate determination of weight loss adequacy. Two key aspects within bariatric treatment include (1) pre-operative weight status and (2) exercise participation.

(A-1) Pre-operative weight status

Heavier individuals possess greater potential for achieving more weight loss. The premise for this occurrence lies in the fact that more calories exist to be expended from extra body weight. For instance, providing the same daily calories to individuals who vary in weight by fifty, seventy-five, or even one hundred pounds, will always create a greater deficit between the caloric needs of the heavier individual than those of an individual who has less reserve of excess body weight.

Although increased excess body stores will potentially lead to an overall greater weight loss, formulas have been created to denote an even more important measurement within the obese population—"Significance of Weight Loss."

Significance of weight loss success is based upon *Percentage of Excess Body Weight Loss (EBWL%)*. EBWL% is = *Weight loss / Total Excess Weight*.

The standard rate of success for bariatric surgery has been designated as a minimum of 50 percent (EBWL), which is maintained for five or more years. Current statistics report a 64 percent success rate based on this standard.[1]

Before determining EBWL%, *Total Excess Weight* must be calculated from the difference between *Pre-operative Weight Status and Ideal Weight*.

For example, someone weighing 250 pounds with an ideal weight of 135 is carrying a total excess weight of 115 pounds. This individual lost 100 pounds, bringing his/her weight down to 150 pounds. Calculate the percentage of excess body weight loss, by dividing 100 by 115 for an EBWL of 87(%). Eighty-seven percent of EBWL is an excellent achievement. Furthermore, sustaining this level of weight loss for greater than five years would yield a very successful surgical outcome as recognized by the bariatric medical field.

(A-2) Exercise participation

After years of studying the metabolic phenomena, it is without question that calories will be lost to energy production when expenditure exceeds intake. The opposite is also true in that calories will accumulate into stored energy when intake exceeds expenditure. This is why participation in a suitable exercise regimen is such an essential factor to achieving optimal weight loss success, regardless of the course of weight loss treatment, bariatric or traditional.

When assessing weight loss, it is both necessary and beneficial to determine what extent the patient is exercising. If it is concluded that the patient is not exercising, then a fitness evaluation should be performed to rule out any physical and/or orthopedic contraindications. If inactivity is caused by a lack of motivation or a lack of availability to an appropriate facility or home equipment, then alternative solutions should be developed with the patient.

For many obese individuals, the only type of exercise that can be performed comfortably without experiencing orthopedic pain is non-weight bearing activities such as, aquatics and bicycling. If walking is an option, then encouragement should be given to performing this activity, since walking is the most natural form of body movement, not to mention that greater caloric expenditure is achieved when performing weight-bearing activities.

(B) A second factor to consider before given an adjustment relates to inadequacy of satiation during a meal along with inadequate satiety between meals.

Satiation is the feeling experienced when hunger is no longer present. Eating in a state where hunger is not the driving force, has the potential in and of itself to limit the intake of calories. Individuals living with disordered eating behaviors are typically not able to engage internal cues of satiation to help determine appropriate intake levels. With the band helping to restrict the physical intake of food, recipients of this tool have the opportunity to learn positive habits based on internally driven cues of satiation.

Due to the restrictive nature of band surgery, it is quite common for patients to eat past the point of satiation because of pre-established disordered eating behaviors such as eating until uncomfortably full. Patients are, therefore, always encouraged to try and consciously eat to a level of "comfortable satisfaction" after banding surgery. Comfortable satisfaction of intake is noted as a feeling of consuming just enough food to eliminate feelings of hunger- that is it! Once hunger is eliminated, no additional food should be consumed.

Consuming food to a level associated with uncomfortable physical fullness is never recommended after surgery due to the negative physical and psychological effects that can occur. The negative physical effects include intense pain in the upper stomach area, regurgitation, and/or vomiting. Unhealthy psychological effects, such as a diminished internal awareness of food consumption, are often associated with eating to a level that produces physical discomfort.

Satiety, in comparison to satiation, develops after food has been ingested. Satiety delays the onset of the next meal and can reduce total food consumption at the next meal as well. Those living with the band experience enhanced satiety when eating the highest quality foods. High quality foods help retain fullness after the meal is well completed because they are slower to flow out of the pouch and down into the stomach. The trickle effect of food dissipating from the pouch helps reduce the appetite to an appropriate metabolic level. Without the common plague of intense fluctuations in appetite, banded patients can eliminate unnecessary caloric intake between meals.

Following Lap-Band surgery, eating lean protein foods in combination with vegetables (lean and green) will enhance feelings of both satiation and satiety. Satiation is enhanced and satiety is prolonged because foods of dense protein and vegetable content have the capacity to distend the pouch maximally while also remaining within the pouch for an extended time. Maximal distention of the pouch will send signals to the brain that satiation is achieved. Furthermore, keeping the pouch distended with food will provide a continuous feedback to the nerves residing in the brain. This entire process is what promotes adequate satisfaction of intake while consuming smaller portions and fewer calories. Once food has left the pouch to enter the remaining lower part of the stomach (where food begins to disseminate by normal digestive processes), feelings of hunger can quickly resume because the pouch will no longer be distended to prolong satiety.

1.   Deitel, M., 2003.

Factors Known to Influence Lap-Band Adjustments

The process for obtaining adjustments are dependent upon factors that are both standard to the Lap-Band, as well as, variables that are patient specific. Universal standards governing adjustments include the type and size of the band. Since approval of the original Lap-Band in 2001, bands of different diameters have been developed to meet the unique anatomical features of every recipient. There are currently two different systems used with the laparoscopic adjustable gastric banding procedures, The Lap-Band System (Allergan recently purchased the rights to the Lap-Band System from Inamed) and The Realize Band. In order to develop a general understanding related to the adjustment process of your band it would be advantageous for you to know which Lap-Band you have. Check with your bariatric surgeon as to the type and the size of the band that he/she has given to you.

Two key factors specific to the patient receiving an adjustment include his/her perceived degree of food restriction and existing tolerance to the most preferred band-friendly foods.

The level of physical restriction created by the "unfilled" band is unique to every patient. Although the unfilled band creates a certain degree of restriction, consumption capacity will quite possibly be more than anticipated because the band has not yet been adjusted to meet the needs of that specific recipient. While some experience severe to moderate restriction, most individuals report mild to insignificant restriction of food intake. This is why 90 to 95 percent of Lap-Band recipients will endure a series of adjustments until their band has reached a level of what is commonly referred to as the "sweet spot." The sweet spot is associated with tolerating a reasonable assortment of high-quality foods at a quantity that is both satisfying and nourishing. The remaining population (5 to 10 percent) will never require an adjustment because of the effective degree of restriction exerted purely from the unfilled band.

Failure to execute favorable behaviors surrounding food intake may prevent or delay adjustments. If an individual experiences painful discomfort or recurrent episodes of regurgitation and/or vomiting, an adjustment should be postponed until difficulties with ingestion improve. It is extremely important that patients are able to consume meals at a slow pace to allow for the breakdown of food to a mushy consistency before swallowing. Making this a consistent daily habit will ensure optimal tolerance to food. It is not advisable to create a smaller opening between the pouch and lower stomach if the patient is displaying poor food tolerance. Adjusting to a level of severe restriction too quickly can manifest time-consuming medical care along with possible psychological difficulty. Care would be needed to re-adjust the level of restriction by aspirating saline from inside the band so food tolerance and adequacy of intake can improve. Psychologically, patients can experience trouble adjusting appropriately to the restriction of the band (regardless of the degree) when adjustments are initially too aggressive. From a behavioral perspective, it is therefore strongly recommended to administer the saline restriction in small, multiple increments to allow adequate time for appropriate adaptation. Adaptation will need to be made with regard to chewing, pace of consumption, and at times even modifying the texture of food.

Once adequate mastication (chewing) of food is regularly performed, adjustments can be granted at appropriate intervals throughout one's weight loss journey. Adjustments will occlude the opening to where food passes. Modifying the opening to a reduced level will promote reduction of intake with prolonged fullness. Similar to a time-released capsule, food will slowly dissipate through the upper pouch and into the lower stomach, thus helping to suppress hunger both during and after the conclusion of the meal.

An overall greater number of adjustments are provided during the first year in living with the band than obtained during any other time after surgery. This appears to be the case because patients have shown to take a keen interest initially following surgery in obtaining the advisable progression of physical restriction so weight loss can occur at an appropriate rate. Typically, women need four to five adjustments within the first year. Men on the other hand, do well with approximately two to three adjustments. The differentiation between genders appears to be related to anatomical features (men typically are internally larger than women are) and choices of food (men commonly consume foods that are of more solid density (e.g., meats)—where women tend to favor breads and other soft density carbohydrate-based food, (which help to stabilize hormones and their affect on serotonin). Once again, adjustments will vary in number depending not only on the individual as it relates to food choices and habits of intake, but also based on the size and type of band provided.

There is believed to be a state of natural osmosis, which reduces the saline residing in the band over an extended period post-operatively. Restriction within the band may unexpectedly feel significantly less following substantial weight reduction. When weight loss occurs at a very significant level, not only is weight reduced from external areas of the body (waist, hips, legs, etc.), but also internally as well (specifically surrounding the organs (e.g., the stomach). This loss of fat tissue will obviously reduce the restriction of the band since the band is placed around the upper part of the stomach. It is therefore advised to revisit your bariatric practice following significant weight loss to evaluate the restrictive capacity of the band.

Factors Known to Influence the Rate of Saline Administered at Each Adjustment

The amount of saline given for each adjustment is dependent initially on the internal circumference of the band. Presently, Allergan has four-patented Lap-Band's available to patients. Ethicon, a division of Johnson and Johnson, was granted (November 2007) the rights to distribute the Realize Band. Bands of variable size have been created to accommodate the broad range of individual anatomical features.

During pre-operative meetings, the bariatric surgeon will educate the patient as to which band(s) he/she is most comfortable utilizing in their operating room. The type and size of the band will be determined once surgery is initiated. Upon initiation of surgery, the surgeon will be able to obtain a first-hand assessment as to which band will allow for the best fit. Of the bands available, it is ultimately the surgeon's decision to decide which band fits best for the patient.

As a patient then proceeds for follow-up treatment, assessments will be conducted to determine the need for an adjustment. The need for an adjustment is based upon success in weight loss, tolerance to foods of highest quality and the degree to which liquids are not consumed during or shortly following (one hour) the completion of a meal. Consuming generally more than two ounces (1/4 cup) of water during and shortly after meals will reduce the beneficial effects of surgery—to attain and remain comfortably satiated several hours following the completion of a small to moderate quantity of food. Even more importantly, consideration of an adjustment is strongly determined by the extent to which satiation is achieved when eating a meal followed by the length of time that satiety is maintained once the meal is completed.

If the need presents, saline will be provided in a given number of ccs of solution. The amount of saline provided is highly dependent upon which band was surgical implanted. A band with a smaller surface area will require less saline to restrict the internal diameter. Comparatively, a band with a larger surface area will require more saline to restrict the internal diameter. Following an initially designated adjustment, saline is then added in specific increments. Guidelines have been set forth by bariatric medical professionals as to the most effective incremental advances of saline to be given at each adjustment. Bariatric medical practices have these useful guidelines at their disposal for treatment of their patients.

While adjustments are provided on an individual case basis, patients are encouraged to return for follow-up appointments as they see fit until the level of restriction is determined to be optimal, with regard to weight loss goals and tolerance of intake. Allocated time between adjustments varies greatly with each patient due to each individual's perceived degree of restriction. The degree of restriction can be further assessed by means of an objective or subject measurement.

If available, patients may take a barium swallow x-ray to evaluate the flow of liquid through the banded-pouch area and down to the lower stomach. If the flow is very slow and appears significantly delayed, it may indicate an adjustment that is too tight and overly restricted. If on the other hand, the flow is very quick with no apparent "hang-time" from the banded-pouch area, then it may indicate an adjustment that is too loose and not sufficiently restricted. If a barium swallow x-ray is unavailable or impractical to perform, another option includes having the individual drink a beverage of modified thickness with a subjective clinical assessment as to the extent of restriction.

At the start of each adjustment process, it is of pertinence to evaluate the existence and degree of hunger as expressed directly by the patient. If hunger is experienced on a consistent basis, it is important to assess existing eating habits and food choices. Without regular consumption of solid consistency protein and vegetable foods, hunger may not be managed effectively. If good tolerance and frequent consumption of these foods is reported, a greater quantity of fill could bring that individual to the most beneficial level of restriction. On the other hand, poor tolerance to challenging, yet preferred foods (such as white meat chicken and turkey, steak, pork, and vegetables of fibrous texture) would strongly indicate less need for saline and more devotion to executing key intake habits.

It is also of extreme importance to assess the individual's drinking habits, particularly when food is entering the pouch and for a short time after as well. Refraining from drinking during meals and for approximately one hour following a meal is by far one of the most important commitments to effectively utilizing the band's key anatomical restrictive feature. Unfortunately it can also be one of the most challenging habits to modify.

As a society, we generally consume meals in a fashion of "bite and gulp." We take a bite of food, typically very large, followed by an immediate gulp of liquid, which for many people is enhanced in quantity and calories, and is also often carbonated. The problem with this behavior is two-fold for the individual eating with the band. One aspect has to do with executing necessary mechanics of intake including consuming small bites of thoroughly chewed food in a slow manner. The second aspect involves preventing the flush of food quickly through the pouch. Allowing for maximal and prolonged distention of the pouch through a process of 'food accumulation' will promote the highest degree of satiation. In addition, carbonation is not well tolerated, whether in the presence or absence of food because of the expansion of gas in the small stomach pouch. In essence, the biting and gulping habits that allow for the intake of large meals in a very short time period are the exact opposite habits that need to be properly performed following surgical intervention.

On a side note, regardless of living with the band or not, proper digestion of food can only occur through adequate break down in the mouth. When food is not chewed to a mushy consistency, havoc occurs throughout the digestive system. The nutrients obtained from our food cannot be obtained within our cells without first bathing food in the presence of salivary enzymes, which exist in our mouth. The longer we take time to masticate each bite, the better our digestive capacity.

In addition to many behavioral changes required after surgical intervention, not drinking with meals or shortly after will become much easier with time. Remember, the quantity of intake is significantly reduced, thereby making the need for hydration much less, both during and shortly following the meal. If an individual indicates that they have not been compliant with this essential habit, providing strategies to overcome their difficulties would serve them better than providing an adjustment. These strategies include hydrating well between meals, even in small sips immediately before beginning the meal, if that is found to be helpful.

Regardless of when and what steps are taken to receiving appropriate adjustments, a "well" fitted band enables the patient to enjoy a broad range of high-quality foods with adequate tolerance of intake while achieving four to five hours of comfortable satiation between meals. Achieving this goal however requires restructuring old habits through a process of self-discovery. As people discover and gently conform to the habits that will assist in effective use of their tool, long-term commitments are made. These commitments then further expand into a whole array of healthy lifestyle habits. Adjustments are only a part of the process and need to be balanced while living through many experiences with the band.

Preparation Before and After an Adjustment

Before undergoing an adjustment, it is advised to refrain from consuming solid foods for a couple of hours before the procedure. Solid foods remain in the upper pouch for an extended time based on the nature of consistency. Distention in the pouch due to remnants of solid food could present for a more challenging adjustment. If intake is needed within a few hours of an adjustment, full liquids and/or soft, mushy foods are advised. This type of intake will ensure that the upper stomach pouch is completely empty and non-distended at the time of the adjustment.

Full liquid items include yogurt, milk, pudding, and soup. Consideration of caloric content should be given when choosing full liquid items. Consuming low-fat or non-fat full liquid items will allow for reduced caloric consumption. Soft, mushy foods include egg salad and tuna fish, cottage cheese, applesauce, mashed potato, hot cereal, creamed spinach, and butternut squash to name a few.

After obtaining an adjustment, it is important to follow specific intake guidelines. These guidelines include consuming clear and/or full liquids for the first twenty-four hours following the adjustment. A soft, mushy food plan is then recommended for the next forty-eight hours. This advice is provided to ensure optimal tolerance while the recipient becomes familiar with the level of physical restriction imparted by their band.

Upon progression of your dietary intake to the soft, mushy food plan, it is important to make note of your tolerance to these modified consistency foods, as well as, to the quantity that can be comfortably consumed. If soft, mushy foods are providing more than adequate restriction, to the point of not eating a sufficient daily quantity, then progression to solid foods should be delayed for one week. During that one-week period, foods of soft, mushy consistency should be consumed along with occasional full liquids to help meet nutritional needs. This recommendation is made because the adjustment may be temporarily too tight. Continued intake of soft, mushy food is recommended until either ease of consumption improves due to innate flexibility of the adjustment or through creating a wider outlet by removing some saline from the band.

For some unknown medical phenomenon, an adjustment can feel abnormally tight or completely the opposite, too loose for up to two weeks following an adjustment. It is, therefore, advised to slowly progress dietary consistency and return to your medical practice to evaluate the overall adjustment process.

One key aspect of reverting back to full liquids and then soft, mushy food is behavioral adaptation. Consuming a liquid followed by a soft, mushy meal plan before initiating solid foods, will allow time to modify the pace at which meals are consumed. An adjustment is typically provided to restrict the opening between the upper stomach pouch and the remaining lower stomach. This restriction will require a much slower pace of consumption, along with thorough mastication of all food before swallowing, otherwise a greater degree of intolerance can be experienced.

Intolerance is associated with painful ingestion, regurgitation, and/or vomiting. If there is a consistent lack of tolerance to high-quality foods, which is unable to be rectified through improvement of habits, then an assessment should be made pertaining to the degree of restriction. In certain situations, an adjustment may be needed to aspirate saline out of the band to allow for an easier flow of food through the band.

To a certain degree, a wider diameter is counter-productive to the effective use of surgery. A larger opening will not only allow for an enhanced portion of food, but will also reduce satiation. Therefore, executing necessary behavioral changes to allow for tolerance of solid to semi-solid foods is of utmost importance.

Difference of Restriction After Surgery Compared to the Restriction Experienced Following an Adjustment

Patients report a difference in restriction immediately post-surgery compared to the restriction obtained after receiving a fill. We know this to be true because the restriction obtained during the weeks following surgery is due to swelling of tissue surrounding the newly placed band. This swelling provides a definitive physical restriction whereby full-liquid beverages are slow to consume. The occluded opening through the banded area will prevent patients from drinking the recommended liquids at a quick and rapid pace. The intake of liquids must be consumed at a slow pace. Occlusion is only temporary though. Once swelling heals, a mild degree of restriction is provided from the band exclusively. Modification of restriction is then made possible through adjustments or 'fills'.

Following an adjustment or subsequent adjustments, the restriction obtained is still noticeably felt, however, not to the same degree or level that was experienced immediately after surgery. Restriction obtained from the administration of saline into the internal (ballooned) area of the band (hence providing a fill) is intended to provide a moderate level of occlusion. This level of restriction should always allow for the consumption of preferred (solid) foods with consideration given to performing band specific intake habits. Adjustments are not intended to be at an extreme level of tightness (as occurred immediately post-operative, secondary to tissue swelling) because this level of restriction can be structurally harmful to the banded area. In addition, a significantly restricted opening may mandate an exclusive full liquid meal plan because of food intolerance. Trying to consume food when liquids are so challenging, may lead to erratic regurgitation and/or vomiting. Furthermore, not being able to return to eating foods of variable consistency can lead to unfavorable social and psychological ramifications. While waiting to receive an initial adjustment, it is best to remain patient and remember the body is healing from surgery. This is a time to embrace important changes and avoid placing high expectations of weight loss. Weight loss will progressively occur following appropriate adjustments provided in the presence of new, self-serving and healthy food intake habits.

Once making an informed decision to seek surgical weight loss intervention, it is imperative that you begin to make a commitment to take care of yourself not only nutritionally, but also physically and emotionally as well.

Necessary Commitment

Committing to undergo bariatric surgery is unlike any other commitment you have ever made in your life, or for that matter, may ever make again. This well-informed decision implies "conscious choice-making." In every given moment, we have access to an immeasurable number of choices. Often times though, people and circumstances trigger our conditioned reflexes into predictable behavior. Because of such conditioning, we typically engage in repetitive responses to environmental stimuli. Most people commonly fail to remember that they have a choice in every thought or action made at every moment. Simply witnessing the choices we make at the very moment that we make them can be very empowering. This empowerment can influence all areas of our life including how we decide to nourish our body, along with what physical activities we engage in to promote good health.

Your decision to dedicate your way of life to the fundamentals of surgery is a life-long obligation that does not end merely with the attainment of a healthy weight. For as long as you have a surgical mechanism by which to govern your lifestyle, there are essential practices to live by. These practices are commonly classified as habits.

Humans have often been referred to as creatures of "habit." Habits can simply represent a regular tendency or practice that is hard to give up. There are those habits we consider life sustaining and those that we constantly try to modify or change because they do not serve us well.

As compared to your pre-operative lifestyle, there will be necessary habits to develop that will be of tremendous benefit while embarking on your surgical weight loss journey. On the other hand, there will be certain habits that are discouraged because they will not allow you to utilize your surgical tool most effectively.

Although the Lap-Band is intended to work well under the best of surgical implantations, you must not expect the band to provide all the restraint necessary to reach your goals. Placement of the Lap-Band is a significant factor to attaining a healthier weight and living a balanced lifestyle, but the effort required to achieving this new state of wellness begins the moment you take the first step on this journey.

A misconception exists among many uneducated people who believe the band in and of itself will provide all that is needed to obtaining a reduced body weight. The band is not something of a magical phenomenon. The band will not automatically train your mind and body to consume the highest quality foods in the most favorable manner. Successful application of this tool requires dedication to performing specific band-friendly eating patterns!

Nutritional Strategies That Can Help Ensure Adequate Health and Healing After Surgery

1. Reduce the consumption of highly processed foods and those that contain considerable amounts of fat and simple sugars. Foods rich in fat include fried items; snacks such as cookies, cakes, donuts, ice cream, and chips; whole milk, whole cheese, marbled meats, and whole eggs. Foods rich in simple sugar include cookies, cakes, donuts, ice cream, candy, white bread, white rice, white pasta, and refined cereals.

2. Focus on eating lean protein at every meal. Foods rich in lean protein include chicken, fish, turkey, beef, tuna fish, egg (whites and/or beaters), beans, soy products (e.g., tofu and tempeh), low-fat sliced cheese, ricotta, and cottage cheese.

3. Experiment with adding a variety of fresh fruits and fresh vegetables to your dietary regimen.

4. Be sure to drink at least 64 ounces of water each day.

5. Start to eliminate beverages that contain carbonation and calories.

6. Supplement your daily intake with a chewable, powder or liquid multivitamin-mineral formula.

Behavioral Strategies That Can Help With Adjusting to Surgically Imposed Restriction

1. Plan your daily meal schedule. Consider what your responsibilities are for the day and make a "game plan" outlining the best time and place for consuming your meals. Then answer the following questions.

   - How much time do you have allotted for each meal?
   - Is that enough time to enjoy your eating experience?
   - If not, how can you manage your time more effectively to allow the opportunity to encompass your total well being (body, mind, and spirit) while consuming your meal?

2. Pay attention to emotionally driven eating tendencies such as eating when feeling bored, anxious, upset, frustrated, or even during times of happiness. The first step in modifying non-hunger related eating habits is to bring awareness to your actions. Effective action-changing strategies can then be developed.

3. Focus on eating when you are only feeling physically hungry. To do so, try listening to internal cues such as "true belly" hunger. Many people who struggle in weight eat to prevent hunger because it can feel overwhelmingly uncomfortable. Being able to recognize comfortable, physical hunger is a positive aspect to eating from a place of internal awareness.

4. Avoid multitasking while eating. Do not eat while: watching television, reading, using the computer, talking on the telephone, driving an automobile, or when distracted by any means.

5. Create a peaceful atmosphere for mealtime. Remove clutter from the table and use soft lighting and soothing music in the background, especially if dining alone.

6. Sit with your back in an upright and straight position while focusing on chewing thoroughly and tasting each mouthful.

7. Set a timer for fifteen to twenty minutes at each meal.

8. Identify how hungry you feel before starting your meal. On a scale of 1 to 10, with 1 = extreme hunger, 5 = moderate hunger, and 10 = no sense of hunger, what number would you use to signify your hunger level? If eating at a level of 1 to 4, try to identify factors related to feeling so hungry (e.g., too many hours between meals, low quality food choices at prior meal). If eating at a level (in the opposite direction) of 9 to 10, try again and identify factors that have prompted a desire for food without the presence of physical hunger (e.g., boredom, anxiety, emotional distress).

9. Place your food on a smaller plate and eat with smaller utensils (e.g., baby forks or spoons or unfamiliar eating tools such as chopsticks) to enhance sensitivity to reduced portions.

10. Try eating with your non-dominate hand to facilitate a slow pace of intake.

11. Place your utensil down between each bite of food and remove your hands from the table (i.e., place hands in your lap or under your leg).

12. Chew food slowly. Concentrate on chewing all food until it feels mushy in your mouth before swallowing. It is suggested to chew each mouthful for up to thirty times before swallowing!!! When food is properly chewed in this manner, the beginning stages of digestion can occur within the mouth.

13. Avoid carbonated, calorie containing, and iced beverages (including iced water) along with hot drinks during meals. It is best only to sip, if needed, room temperature water while eating.

14. Observe how much liquid you drink while eating. Recognize if you are drinking because you feel thirsty or to enhance the quantity of your meal.

15. Recognize how you feel as you consume your meal. Assess if you are beginning to feel comfortably satisfied before completing the remaining food on your plate. How would you describe feeling comfortably satisfied?

16. Try to end your meal before feeling full and/or physically uncomfortable.

17. Observe how much liquid you drink within the first hour after completing your meal.

18. Monitor your rate of satisfaction and return of physical hunger after each meal. Did you snack between any meals? If so, at what time? What did you choose for a snack? Identify how hungry you felt before eating your snack. On a scale of 1 to 10, with 1 = extreme hunger, 5 = moderate hunger and 10 = no sense of hunger. What number would you use to signify your appetite? If snacking at a level of 9 to 10, try indentifying factors related to your habits of intake (e.g., feeling emotionally unstable, anxious, stressed, or possibly just been exposed to foods that were appealing to your taste buds, smell, and sight).

Mental Strategies That Can Help With Emotionally Adjusting to Surgical Intervention

1. First, accept the fact that your Lap-Band is simply a "tool". This tool is designed to provide a "mechanical impediment" that will alleviate hunger and elevate satiety while eating a reduced quantity of food. Therefore, you must be accountable for executing behaviors that will facilitate proper use of your surgical tool. Failure to acknowledge the Lap-Band as a tool will displace responsibility on the surgery, and not where it should be, within the person who utilizes it. Due to the underlying surgical premise, which is to provide a physical entity to modify behavioral and emotional issues surrounding food favorably, it would only be a disservice to the recipient if he or she fails to connect with their Lap-Band as being a tool.

2. Dissolve all previous failed attempts with implementing externally focused weight loss programs. Externally based dieting regimens emphasize restricting food while controlling the quality of intake. On a whole, use of these external directives has failed to help individuals eat in response to physiological hunger and satiety cues.

    Conceptually speaking, dieting is an external process that requires the individual to disassociate from internal cues. At its most extreme, dieting totally removes any personal connection with internal signals. Internal signals are intended to govern behavior. Unmistakably, dieting teaches one to ignore their hunger. Following this type of restricted, deprivation regimen leads to the development of hunger intolerance, overeating, eating in response to emotions, and ultimately a vicious cycle of poor weight management.

    Various traditional and commercial programs alike recommend a treatment plan based solely on externally controllable sources such as reducing calories, eliminating a specific nutrient (e.g., no carbohydrates but all the protein and fat one can eat), or even food combining (e.g., vegetables can be consumed with either all carbohydrate-based foods or all foods rich in protein). These programs fail to take into consideration the physiological needs of the individual. When placing the control on an entity outside the individual's control, permanent change will no longer exist once deviation from the plan occurs.

Surgery is a completely different realm of treatment. Surgical intervention allows for reconnecting, interpreting, and responding appropriately to internal signals. Through a newly acquired ability, one can reestablish the fundamentals of choosing foods that will replenish metabolic needs without solely basing food selection on a particular diet plan. Eliminating certain foods or following a specific post-banded food regimen will not be encouraged for the most part, however, fundamental nutrition principles are essential to ensure good health and overall well-being.

3. Was there an emotional connection to any meal or snack intake? For example, did you choose to eat because you were feeling bored, frustrated, angry, happy, or even excited? If yes, consider journal writing to identify possible underlying emotions that provoked a desire to eat. In turn, start to focus on developing positive non-eating behaviors to help deal with those emotions.

Journal Writing Ideas

a. Thoughts leading up to intake

b. Circumstances leading up to intake

c. Time and place

d. With whom

e. Time of last intake

f. Content and quantity of prior consumption

g. Level of appetite at the start of intake

h. Level of satiation at the completion of intake

i. Content & quantity of current consumption

j. Feelings associated with foods chosen

k. Feelings associated with the quantity consumed

Developing Key Eating Patterns Will Help Optimize the Effective Use of the Lap-Band Tool

These eating patterns include:

1. Consume your first intake of the day within two hours of awakening.
2. When consuming solid foods, schedule three meals (one every five hours) daily, along with one healthy snack, as needed.
3. Eat meals within a non-distracted environment.
4. Take twenty minutes to consume a balanced, nourishing meal.
5. Learn to chew all food to a mushy consistency before swallowing.
6. Eat to nourish the body and drink to hydrate the body; however avoid eating and drinking simultaneously.
7. Choose foods that are rich in nutrients such as protein and vegetables (lean and green).
8. Choose protein foods and vegetables that are of solid texture.
9. Eat protein foods first followed by a vegetable and then consume a starch food at the very end of each meal.
10. Discover physically connected eating techniques.

1. Consume your first meal of the day within two hours of awakening.

Positive eating patterns begin first thing in the morning with breakfast. Failure to consume a nourishing breakfast meal within two hours of beginning your day, can not only diminish metabolism, but also surprisingly with the band, it can lead to the possibility of poorly tolerating food for the remainder of the day. Breakfast is just as the name implies, *break* the *fast*, which has come to be of even more significance amongst those individuals with the band. It is of extreme importance to avoid postponing your first meal of the day beyond the first two hours.

Our metabolism generates its starting fuel from the food we consume. Without consuming enough overall basic nutrients throughout the day, fewer calories will be needed to fuel the body. It is similar to a fire; we need to feed the fire (logs and wood) in order for the fire to continue burning a flame of heat (energy).

The importance of breakfast intake for surgical patients goes even far beyond satisfying metabolic needs. There has been a common link between the omission of breakfast and poor food tolerance amongst those who have had restrictive, banding surgery. Patients often describe experiencing unusual "tightness" of the band when food is not consumed within a reasonable time after awakening. Restricted afternoon intake also is frequently experienced when breakfast is not consumed until many hours after beginning the day.

The exact mechanism for this phenomenon is still unknown; however, it is hypothesized that the area where the band lies can become more restricted if fasting occurs for an extended length of time. Restriction could be caused by unidentified spasms of the lower esophagus and upper stomach—the exact area where the band lies. This effect can occur regardless of the time of day in which fasting has taken place. It is quite possible for patients to experience this phenomenon as an overnight fast because it is often challenging to consume breakfast regularly due to difficulties with time management and limitations in the physiological need for calories.

For instance, eating at seven in the evening and not eating again until noon the next day would leave a total of seventeen hours without the intake of anything greater than the consistency of water. For a banded person, this lengthy fasting could make the area where food passes extremely occluded; the greater the occlusion, the smaller the opening and the increase in possibility for intolerance.

When lunch is difficult to consume due to the absence of breakfast, patients may choose to eat mushy foods or even drink liquids as their meal. Although tolerance to mushy foods and beverages is a better choice due to the lack of texture and subsequently an easier flow through the obstructed opening; sustained satiety will not occur. Onset of early hunger could then lead to the intake of excess calories.

2. When consuming solid foods, schedule three meals (one every five hours) daily, along with a one healthy snack, as needed.

During the early post-operative period, patients are instructed to consume six, small meals daily to provide for adequate nourishment without endangering the pouch by consuming too great of a quantity at one time. Furthermore, it is recommended to consume a meal every two to three hours to ensure the intake of six meals throughout the day.

The exact timing of meals should be individualized to meet the person's daily sleep and activity patterns. For example, there may be a period in the day where the activity performed is more physical, thus expending more calories. If this were to occur, spacing meals two hours apart instead of three would be more beneficial. At other times, sedentary activities may be occurring, and waiting three hours as opposed to two would essentially be more beneficial. Consideration to the timing of meals post-banded is considered to be invaluable, however in order to take full advantage of the guidelines, it must be in accordance with one's lifestyle.

The early post-operative period entails a full-liquid plan for approximately two weeks followed by a soft-mushy food phase for an additional two weeks. Due to the consistency of full liquids and soft-mushy foods, fullness would not normally extend for any great length of time. However, due to the prominent swelling surrounding the opening where the Lap-Band resides, in combination with the intake of a meal every two to three hours, short-term satiety is highly achievable. This has proven to be true in many cases of early post-operative patients, as they have reported a physical inability to consume all six meals. If this happens to occur infrequently (no more than two to three times in a week where one to two meals were not taken), then nutritional adequacy would not be of significant concern. If on the other hand, more frequent omission of meals occurred (more than four times in a week where two to three meals were not taken), then you should discuss this with your bariatric physician and/or nutritionist to ensure the attainment of adequate macronutrients. Attaining adequate nourishment can be managed by varying choices of supplements, quantity of intake and/or timing of intake.

Once solid foods are introduced following a four-week post-operative period, it is then recommended to resume a three-meal-a-day pattern with an optional healthy snack (or what may be referred to as a mini-meal, which is half the quantity of a regular meal), depending on daily energy expenditure. With the consumption of solid foods, satiety will be prolonged because of the "textured" food consistency. In addition, quantity of intake is enhanced; therefore consuming a meal every five hours is a more appropriate period for a daily pattern of three solid meals. Be mindful that waiting longer than five hours is not recommended because one's appetite will enhance, which then can lead to poor intake habits.

3. Eat meals within a non-distracted environment.

Partaking in any other activity while consuming a meal will limit intuitive eating awareness (IEA). IEA is the ability to instinctively recognize and acknowledge body-mind interrelatedness. IEA does not end at that point however. It further entails an appropriate response to that awareness, which would require an action to either (a) stop eating or (b) continue consuming food based on the premise that internal hunger is still present.

As food enters the pouch, physical distention of the newly created "stomach area" will trigger the brain and allow for mental recognition. The moment at which attention is no longer given to the intake of food, physical and mental connections will be lost. Like telephone wires being crossed, which causes the conversation to become muffled and incomprehensive, your body is experiencing the same lack of communication. This is why fully focused attention must be given at all meals otherwise, communication between the body and mind becomes disconnected. Band treatment will help to reestablish this connection, but only in an environment that honors the link between physical and psychological recognition.

Individuals must be motivated and willing to do their best to treat their eating disorder from internal awareness. Internal regulation will require controlling for external factors as well. It is highly recommended to eliminate performing all activities when eating, such as watching television, driving a vehicle, answering the telephone, working on the computer, reading, or even care taking of another individual - all of which to some degree requires attention. Upon the intake of meals, try simply to enjoy the company you are in (even when dining alone, enjoy being with yourself) and soak in the flavor, aroma, and texture of the food that is on your plate.

Begin each meal by taking a few deep breathes to help clear your mind while reducing any stress or anxiety you may be feeling. There is a strong belief within bariatric medicine that feelings of stress and/or anxiety can lead to poor tolerance of food, regardless of the habits performed while eating. Although there is no scientific evidence to justify this problematic intolerance to food, it is believed to be the result of spasms radiating at the junction of the esophagus and stomach, the exact location of the band. For instance, even if someone made a conscious effort to consume his or her meal in an optimal manner (slow pace and full mastication of food while enjoying his or her intake in a relaxed environment), intolerance can still occur due to internal stress that resides within the individual. Therefore, developing stress-relieving techniques can help to optimize food tolerance following Lap-Band surgery.

Everyone is unique in areas of stress reduction, however, some basic stress relieving techniques include:

a. Journal writing
b. Stepping outside for a breath of fresh air
c. Taking a walk
d. Visualizing and/or Meditating
e. Calling a friend
f. Listening to music
g. Taking a warm bath
h. Reading something of interest
i. Engaging in a hobby
j. Painting a picture
k. Playing cards
l. Taking a drive in the car
m. Going shopping
n. Having a massage

4. Take twenty minutes to consume a balanced, nourishing meal.

Twenty minutes has been designated as the ideal period for completing a meal following surgery. This period has been recommended for two main reasons.

One reason involves the consistency of food. Solid food is highly preferred, which will assist in experiencing early onset satiation at the meal along with ensuring post-meal satiety. Consuming solid food will require extensive chewing to promote good tolerance. If soft-mushy foods were chosen, then less time will be required to complete the meal due to limited chewing. Soft-mushy food will undoubtedly result in less physical restriction and a shorter period of satiety.

A second reason twenty minutes is highly recommended relates to the time needed for the nerves that reside within the brain to recognize and signal comfortable satiation. Inadequate time could lead to uncomfortable fullness, as the nerves of satiation will not be able to send a signal to the brain in such a short time period. This associated uncomfortable feeling of fullness could further lead to painful discomfort.

Discomfort from eating too quickly is not only discouraged from a surgical standpoint, but it will also limit the opportunity to fill the pouch adequately so that prolonged satiety can be experienced. Once discomfort dissipates, there is no associated feeling of satiety because the optimal level of intake was never fully achieved. Therefore, eating too quickly and feeling uncomfortable will tend to produce post-meal hunger much sooner.

The busyness of our lives combined with enormous multitasking will lead most people to eat meals at a less than optimal pace. This behavior will prevent adequate food breakdown, which will inevitably cause some degree of intolerance. In addition, a smaller quantity of food is consumed because of the shorter length of time allocated to complete the meal. Consequently, optimal satiety will not be achieved and hunger can return much earlier than desired.

Long-term satiety can only be achieved when sufficient time is set aside for the enjoyment of meals. Achieving a level of comfortable satiation at mealtime is the primary goal when eating after surgery. Eating to this level is a foreign concept for most weight challenged individuals. Post-banded patients report a deeper understanding of this concept as a result of positive inter-meal feedback from their surgical tool. Comfortable satiation is a feeling that is intended to remain with the individual several hours after intake, thus helping to limit between meal snacking.

There may be those after surgery who feel the need to take an extended period of time to consume a meal because of the belief that "longer is better." Remember the main goal with restrictive, Lap-Band surgery is to enable the individual not only to consume less food at one time, but also to remain well satiated long after a meal is completed. Effective satiation will be reduced when taking longer than thirty minutes (beginning to end) to consume a meal.

When a meal is consumed over a prolonged period of time (thirty minutes or longer), the food consumed at the very beginning of the meal will make its way through the upper pouch and into the lower remaining part of the stomach to begin partial digestion. As one continues to eat, the same cycle occurs where food consumed previously leaves the upper pouch at a quick rate without necessarily filling that intended area all at once. It is always best to eat a given quantity of food at one interval so that the pouch can fully distend while triggering the highest level of satiation. When a banded individual continues to eat a meal after twenty minutes that individual is considered to be consuming a whole separate, second meal. Being consciously aware during the twenty minutes it takes to consume your intake will help to enjoy eating only one meal at a time.

5. Learn to chew all food to a mushy consistency before swallowing.

Swallowing a piece of food that is larger than the opening of where the band sits can lead to discomfort, pain, and/or regurgitation. It is imperative to chew all food adequately before swallowing, especially those of tough texture, including protein enriched foods and fibrous vegetables. Failure to tolerate foods of highest preference (i.e., solid lean protein and solid consistency vegetables) will not only lead to the risk of malnutrition, but it may also promote the intake of slippery foods, which can lead to excessive caloric intake due poor quality food choices and/or the ease of food consumption.

Take for example the scenario of having a poor episode with tolerating baked chicken and steamed broccoli. After the episode has subsided, one may resort to eating chips, cookies, or ice cream given the fact that these foods take limited time and effort to break-down while also being associated with minimal to no risk of poor tolerance.

In addition, consistent poor tolerance to specific foods can cause a long-term psychological "block," not to mention structural damage to the banded site. Feelings of anxiety often develop when eating foods that have caused some prior level of difficulty. Anxiety can then cause spasms to occur around the band, making it more and more difficult to tolerate the food regardless of the way the food was consumed. It is always best to avoid eating a food for approximately one month if poor tolerance has been greatly noted. During that thirty-day period, a psychological separation from the food and poor behavioral tolerance can occur. When the food is then reintroduced, tolerance could significantly improve from the basis of developing a more positive mental outlook.

6. Eat to nourish the body and drink to hydrate the body; however avoid eating and drinking simultaneously.

Obtaining adequate daily hydration is essential to weight loss success, however it is not recommended to drink fluids both during and for one hour following meals. Failure to acclimate to this fluid habit will lead to unfavorable effects.

One such effect is mistakenly distending the stomach pouch with liquid rather solid food. Distention from water consumption will only create a mild and brief modification in appetite. Filling the pouch with food to a level of comfortable distention will produce a feeling of prolonged satiation. Drinking and eating simultaneously can also cause intolerable pressure in the pouch, which can then force food to be regurgitated.

A significant benefit of not drinking while eating lies in the potential to masticate food fully with the help of the salivary glands. Not drinking while eating, creates less tendency to "wash back" food in the mouth, which can lead to a quicker passage through the back of the throat and down the esophagus. If this were to occur, intolerance is more likely, as well as, a larger consumption capacity.

Drinking within one hour following a meal will reduce the post-meal satiety effect of the Lap-Band surgical tool. Liquid mixed with food will soften the consistency, thus allowing food to pass through the upper stomach pouch at a quicker rate. Remember, once the stomach pouch is empty and non-distended, there will be a loss of satiety and a return to hunger sooner.

Consideration should also be given to reducing liquid consumption approximately fifteen minutes before the start of each meal. Consumption of small sips of water before the meal is certainly fine; however taking more than approximately two ounces is not advised. By following this guideline, the possibility of sensing "pseudo" fullness, which is created by fluid rushing into the pouch at a quick rate and temporarily distending the pouch, will be reduced. This will also allow for the development of an appropriate level of hunger to occur before the beginning of the next meal. Additionally, small sips of water can be consumed at a meal or during the hour following a meal as needed to alleviate excessive thirst and/or an inability to comfortably swallow food.

7. Choose foods that are rich in nutrients such as protein and vegetables (lean and green).

When making food choices after surgery, it is important to be consciously aware of the nutritional density obtained from your selection. Restrictive surgery is intended to offer just that, restriction of intake. With quantity of intake reduced to a modified level, quality of food choices become of imperative concern. Reducing the quantity of food requires a conscious effort to choose items that are rich in protein, vitamins, and minerals—the building blocks of a healthful existence; otherwise, malnutrition can be troublesome.

8. Choose protein foods and vegetables that are of solid to semi-solid texture.

Quality of food choices is one of the key considerations when planning meals post-surgery. Another major consideration is "food texture." Choosing food of the highest quality will allow for making the most out of one's intake by conserving calories, whereby choosing food of solid (dense) texture will allow for profound satiation both during and after meals as well.

Foods of solid consistency should be chosen most often. Foods of solid consistency remain in the upper stomach pouch longer due to a heavier consistency. If there is a choice to have a soft-mushy food at a meal, consideration must be given to the remaining foods. It is extremely beneficial to consume at least one solid consistency food at each meal. With the intake of at least one solid food at a meal, satiation will be more easily recognized.

For example, if flaky (e.g., flounder) fish where chosen at a meal for beneficial protein, then the second item should be a minimally steamed vegetable item, such as broccoli, rather than a mushy vegetable, such as creamed spinach. Eating two soft-mushy foods (flounder and creamed spinach) will pass through the pouch quicker without optimizing satiation. To optimize satiation while consuming selective soft-mushy foods, one solid food must also be consumed at the same meal. Additionally, it is recommended to consume the solid food first so that the passage of the soft-mushy food through the pouch is slower.

In comparison, choosing white meat chicken (tougher texture) in place of fish would make it more favorable for the intake of a mushy vegetable like creamed spinach. However, the most beneficial choices to ensure satiety would be white meat chicken and minimally steamed broccoli. Both foods are of solid texture, thereby allowing the stomach pouch to be distended for a longer period of time.

9. Eat protein foods first followed by a vegetable and then consume a starch food at the very end of each meal.

It is essential to consume a protein source in its entirety followed by a vegetable. If then tolerated, a very small portion of a starchy (carbohydrate-rich) food can be consumed to help bring the meal into nutritional balance. If a vegetable is not desired, it is recommended to enhance the quantity of your protein source, rather than intake more carbohydrate-rich foods. By eating foods in this sequence, macronutrient sufficiency, which is needed for a host of metabolic processes including muscle retention, proficient metabolism, proper functioning of organs and adequacy of cellular turnover for healthy skin and hair can be assured. Additionally, consumption of protein and vegetable-based foods will also initiate intra-meal satiation with continued post-meal satiety.

Eating starch-based foods (e.g., bread, pasta, rice and potato) as the last item at meals will help reduce the consumption of easily obtainable calories. Starch-based foods slip through the pouch with less restriction, thereby diminishing satiation and leading to the possibility for over consumption. In addition, for many individuals, carbohydrate-rich foods may over expand once settling into the pouch. Expansion can be very painful with the possibility of experiencing uncomfortable regurgitation.

To reduce intolerance of foods that have a tendency to expand, try these modifications:

1. Foods requiring the process of cooking in water are typically better tolerated when cooked to a mushy consistency rather than al dente.
2. Bread products are better tolerated when toasted because it helps reduce the doughy texture, which can exhibit a sponge effect once settling in the pouch.

It is important to pay attention to the fact that modification of carbohydrate-foods may promote better tolerance of intake, but it also can lead to a greater capacity to eat more. Therefore, portion control techniques must be instituted when eating foods that are rich in carbohydrate, especially when modified in some capacity to enhance tolerance.

As a final note: If there is an occasion for example, where only starch foods are being served (e.g., Italian restaurant) or may be the only food desired, then by all means enjoy your intake, however just be aware of the diminished effect in reaching adequate fullness, as well as post-meal satiety.

10. Discover physically connected eating techniques.

Becoming physically connected with the food you consume represents an inner ability to eat when first feeling physiologically hungry and stopping when initially satisfied. It is a reconnection with the innate ability to consume just enough food to sustain comfortable satiation and then reaching the next meal at a preferred level of hunger. Individuals who have encountered weight difficulties are often genetically unequipped in making that physical connection, as a result of a physiological defect. This physical defect limits the clarity necessary to determine when comfortable satiation is achieved. As a result of this physiological deficit, consistent over consumption manifests various levels of poor weight management.

Lap-Band surgery will provide a physical element to assist in making the body-mind connection, however fully focused attention must be given at each meal in order to truly "own" that benefit. Reconnecting with physically censored habits often promotes choosing foods that are wholesome, satisfying, and health enhancing.

Realistic Expectations

It is only human nature to develop expectations when one has a vested interest in achieving a desired outcome. Motivation to follow through with a specific action or behavior is often driven by "what can I expect to be the end result." Developing a foundation of realistic, achievable expectations can help prevent shortcomings to attaining ones' goals.

Expectations commonly associated with Lap-Band surgery can be collectively categorized within the following areas:

1. Weight Loss
2. Tolerance verse Intolerance of Food
3. Social and Lifestyle Ramifications

1 (A). How much weight can an individual successfully lose?

There are many individual factors that influence quantity of weight loss regardless of the treatment modality. Although factors (such as age, years of weight struggle, genetic predisposition, and activity level) still remain strong determinants of the results following Lap-Band surgical treatment, a standard percentage of success has been designated with this procedure. The standard percentage of success is recognized to be equal to 50 percent of an individual's excess body weight (EBW). Therefore, if someone weighed 100 pounds over their ideal body weight, a loss of 50 pounds would be considered an appropriate standard rate of success.

Success rates have also been classified according to a factor of time. Due to the lack of successful weight loss maintenance by virtually all means of treatment, the bariatric standard of success has been designated as a five-year period. Weight loss occurring during a time period of less than five years does not represent significance in maintenance, which is the most important factor with regards to long-term success. Therefore, if an individual successfully sustained a 50 percent (or greater) loss in excess body weight loss for at least five years, then surgical treatment would prove to be an effective intervention.

Successfully losing 50 percent of one's excess body weight is strongly influenced by the mechanics of the band. These mechanics entail restricting a given quantity of calories on a regular basis while signaling profound satiation. By no means is malabsorption occurring to assist in promoting a greater deficit in caloric consumption. Malabsorption would only occur through procedures that restructure part of the anatomy, as occurs with gastric bypass, for example.

The standard rate of success achieved through more invasive surgeries lies between 70 to 80 percent and in some cases as high as 90 percent. Despite the fact that invasive surgeries present with higher success rates, these percentages appear to occur only initially and not long-term. It has been discovered that maintaining a 50 percent or greater loss in excess weight for five or more years is more often not achieved amongst those patients who have received some form of malabsorptive procedure in treatment of their obesity condition. In essence, surgeries performed with a malabsorptive component, are found to present with weight regain, which thereby reduces the overall rate of success.

A number of factors are related to this faltering success including permanent, unfavorable distention of the stomach pouch, which may in fact be the result of poorly executed intake habits or due to physiological aspects associated with the surgical creation of the stomach pouch. Another prominent reason lies with inappropriate adaptation to post-operative life such as eating non-nourishing foods.

Although the standard rate of success with Lap-Band surgery is less than other invasive surgeries, participating in regular physical activity can certainly enhance weight loss. Increased energy expenditure will help to compensate for the lack of caloric malabsorption. On a positive note, Lap-Band surgery does allow for full nutrient absorption, thereby decreasing the risk of malnutrition and the need for extensive lifelong vitamin-mineral supplementation.

At the other extreme, some may question the possibility of losing too much weight with the help of the band. The probability of this occurring is extremely minimal. The reason this is not typically recognized is because diet induced weight loss is often too difficult to maintain. When weight loss is achieved, energy homeostasis vigorously defends the weight that has been lost through compensatory changes in energy intake and expenditure. Accordingly, efforts to move below a genetically influenced level of body weight are thought to trigger compensatory changes in appetite and energy expenditure that then prevent losing excessive weight.

In addition, the possibility of losing too much weight can be completely avoided by enhancing caloric intake through easily consumable, calorie-enriched liquids. Restriction of the Lap-Band is never occluded to a level that will inhibit the consumption of liquids; therefore, if needed, extra calories can be consumed without difficulty through beverage intake. This is the approach to feeding a growing fetus if in fact a post-banded female where to become pregnant. With pregnancy, complete removal of saline within the band would be performed to allow for additional calories without feeling so satiated.

1 (B). How much time will it take for an individual to successfully reduce their weight to a healthier level?

As mentioned in the previous section, numerous factors influence weight loss, including genetics, pre-existing weight, and weight history along with environmental, behavioral, and psychological issues. Similar to other successfully implemented weight loss modalities, Lap-Band recipients tend to lose considerable weight within a short period of time (first three months) after surgery. At which time, weight loss tends to occur at a slower rate for reasons that are related to metabolic adaptation.

Adaptation to metabolic demands occurs primarily due to a consistently low caloric intake. The body becomes very efficient with expending energy when calories are reduced to a significant level for a prolonged period. In turn, the number of calories needed to carry out bodily demands become much less. When this occurs, weight loss can come to an immediate halt, placing the body into what is referred to as a plateau. A plateau represents an area of stability where what was occurring before based on a given stimulus has now ceased. Plateaus occur naturally (even after undergoing surgical treatment) once the body is physiologically balanced in composition to changes in energy demands.

Small changes in composition of nutrient intake (carbohydrate, protein, and fat) can help stimulate the body's ability to counteract a plateau. However, the underlying resistance to breaking a plateau and losing additional weight lies in the total number of calories. Without utilizing more calories than consumed, plateaus are less resistant to change.

Exercising is strongly encouraged to prevent, or at the very least delay a plateau. Engaging in a personalized exercise regimen where time and effort is devoted to training the body, will greatly assist in breaking through a plateau. There are many different variations of exercise, just as there are many preferences and dislikes amongst people. It would be beneficially self-serving to choose an exercise regimen that fulfills an individual's participation level, as well as one's physical capability. It is also advised for the promotion of long-term adherence to discover a regimen that will provide a sense of personal enjoyment.

Consideration should also be given to the type of exercise performed. The cardiovascular, pulmonary, and skeletal systems receive tremendous benefit from stress-induced exercises that entail steady, rhythmic movements. These movements classify the exercise as aerobic. Aerobic exercises utilize a mixture of fat and carbohydrate nutrients to meet the energy demands of the activity. Aerobic type exercises include, but are not limited to walking, jogging, bicycling, swimming, stair climbing, hiking, and skating.

Due to the variability in exercise participation and its affiliation with plateaus, along with the other patient-specific variables, the estimated time frame to attaining goal weight occurs generally within one to three years. Commitment to a regular (at least three sessions per week for no less than thirty minutes) of physically demanding (mild to moderate intensity) exercise program will help prevent the occurrence of a plateau. Even though weight loss does continue to occur up to the third year post-surgery, considerable success is achieved during the first year. Between the second and third year, weight loss is indeed noted, however, not to the degree that took place throughout the first twelve months.

1 (C). How successful is weight loss maintenance?

Maintenance of weight loss is notably successful not only because of the steady rate at which weight loss occurs, but also because of the following benefits:

a. Adjustability of the Lap-Band
b. Positive behavioral changes that instinctively develop during the early post-operative period

Adjustability of the Lap-Band is a major feature that can be utilized for the life of the band. Obtaining adjustments when deemed necessary will ultimately help to optimize internal regulation. If maintaining a desired body weight becomes more challenging and strategies to modify behaviors favorably and/or food choices have been implemented to the best of one's ability, then additional restriction may further help reduce quantity of intake consumed while sustaining longer post-meal satiety. Remaining in contact with the surgical team members will not only allow for attaining timely adjustments, but it can also have a positive effect with executing beneficial eating behaviors along with guiding an individual's commitment.

Once a desired body weight has been successfully maintained for a considerable period of time (deemed appropriate by the physician and patient), the band can be adjusted in the opposite direction of restriction. Adjustability of the band can always take place in direction of either, inflation or deflation. Adding saline will restrict the opening by inflating the balloon inside the band. In contrast, aspiration of saline will create a larger opening by deflating the balloon residing within the Lap-Band.

Choosing to reduce saline restriction can assist in eating a variety of foods that at one time may have been frustratingly too difficult to tolerate. Having the capability of eating desirable foods without the possibility of intolerance can feel similar to life without the band. However, because the band is still in place, restriction of intake will always be controlled to some extent. Positive transition into long-term use of the band can allow an individual to accept the band as an internal part of their existence. It is important however to make certain that with less restriction there is not a tendency to participate in habits that can jeopardize weight loss success, such as over consuming calorie-rich foods.

Establishing early post-operative changes in eating habits is the second most important factor related to successful weight loss maintenance with the Lap-Band. Radical weight loss surgery involving cutting and stapling of the anatomy (i.e., gastric bypass) curtails intake to such a drastic level (due to the nature of surgery, which creates a tiny stomach pouch with the understanding that over time cell growth will naturally enhance the size of the pouch) that adapting to new eating habits and behaviors are easier to accomplish initially. This is because surgery provides a mechanism which helps establish 'seventy-five percent' of the necessary changes. The remaining twenty-five percent are changes that need to be set-forth and accomplished by the individual.

Committing to such a small percentage of change in the beginning phase of post-surgical intervention is one of the main reasons, in addition to surgical-metabolic adaptation, for late-onset weight regain among gastric bypass recipients. This phenomenon of weight regain within the gastric bypass community typically occurs between the third and fifth year following surgery. Not being able to modify behaviors successfully at the time when surgery provides for maximal physical restriction and malabsorption, is one shortcoming of gastric bypass surgery.

Providing seventy-five percent of the effort toward gaining internal control from surgical intervention may in fact make it more challenging for many bypass patients to commit to the remaining twenty-five percent of effort that they need to apply in order to control for external factors. This responsibility for change is often very difficult and most patients find themselves wrongfully relying on surgical intervention as their sole "tool." By providing a mechanism that requires an even distribution of effort from the controller (i.e., the patient) and the stimulus (i.e., the surgical apparatus), long-term success in behavioral management can be more highly achieved.

Placement of the Lap-Band creates a standard size pouch (larger than the pouch created by stapling and suturing) because cell growth does not enhance the size of the stomach pouch over time. The primary area that can be modified is the opening or outlet for food to travel from the pouch to the remaining lower area of the stomach. Following Lap-Band surgery, fifty percent of the effort to succeed is only possible through the actions of the recipient. The remaining fifty percent is made possible through the effective application of surgery. On a whole, making more of an effort initially in all areas involving food intake will create a more consciously connected adaptation to a long-term, healthier lifestyle.

Lastly, this is another reason for the engagement in an exercise program. Maintaining a reduced body weight can be less difficult when calories are being consistently utilized for movement-generated energy expenditure. Weight challenged individuals possess a reduced metabolic rate compared to individuals of average weight. Therefore, exercising regularly can only serve to enhance the rate at which calories are utilized, thus promoting greater probability in sustaining a reduced body weight.

2 (A). Are there foods that will require a greater level of attentive "mindfulness" with regard to the ease of consumption?

The primary intent of Lap-Band surgery is to modify a given quantity of food. This modification is made possible by the ring-like feature of the band, whose design is to constrict the opening or passageway from the esophagus to the stomach. Similar to the action of a funnel, the passageway will resist the flow of bulky substances (i.e., food of solid consistency). The passageway, however, is unable to produce resistance to substances that are liquid or that turn to a liquid consistency upon ingestion.

For instance; juice, milk, or any other beverage (calorie containing or not) along with yogurt, pudding, ice cream and plain soup (e.g., tomato) will flow at an easier and more rapid rate through the opening to the lower stomach. Once the stomach pouch is no longer holding a substance to keep it distended, hunger can then return within a short period of time. Soups containing some type of food substance (e.g., chicken, turkey, noodles, rice, and vegetables) are found to be of a "chunky" consistency and can slow the rate of displacement from the upper pouch to the lower stomach. This is not to say that plain soups are not advised; it just implies that chunky consistency soups are more apt to promote feelings of satiation.

Examples of food items that liquefy once in contact with salivary and enzymes include chocolate and soft baked products, such as cookies and cakes. Although not of a liquefied consistency initially, these snacks change form upon consumption, thereby, allowing for a greater than average intake without attaining complete satiation.

Another food that liquefies upon ingestion is plain cereal (cereal that does not contain chunky ingredients such as dried fruit, nuts, or clusters). Mixing cereal with milk automatically changes the consistency to mushy and in some instances to a liquefied texture. Mushy or partially liquefied consistency translates into a quicker flow through the opening resulting in a less than optimal feeling of satiation and the possibility of a return to hunger sooner.

A helpful suggestion, which can quite possibly negate the unfavorable effect of consuming foods that liquefy upon intake, is to eat a small quantity of solid consistency food first. Solid food will provide a resistive barrier for the rapid passage of mushy or partially liquefied contents. Applying this pattern of intake will inevitably help reduce the consumption of potentially calorie-rich, non-satiating foods. In turn, desired foods can be consumed, but in a manner that will not contraindicate the use of the band.

When choosing to eat foods that offer limited satiation, it is highly recommended to practice conscious eating techniques. Connecting on a conscious level will help foster-targeted awareness to every aspect associated with the consumption food. This will in essence inhibit the possibility of jeopardizing the use of one's internal tool. Mindful eating techniques involve portioning the quantity of food to be consumed, sitting relaxed in a non-distracted environment, mentally focusing, and most importantly, developing a body-mind connection where taste, flavor, and texture of the food can be fully appreciated. These techniques make it possible to eat a variety of preferred foods while utilizing surgical intervention effectively.

2 (B). Are there foods that will require a greater level of attentive "mindfulness" with regard to difficulty of consumption?

Although there are certain foods that by nature of texture and/or consistency will be more difficult to tolerate, individual differences vary from person to person. Foods that are tolerated well by one individual may not be tolerated well by another. One main reason for the variability in tolerance lies within personal eating habits.

Recommendations to chew food to a mushy consistency can mean different rates of mastication for each and every individual. In addition, there are foods that, despite chewing adequately, can be difficult to consume because of fiber content, chewy-tough texture, or even due to the level in which the food expands upon intake.

Foods associated with high fiber content include, but are not limited to celery, asparagus, broccoli spears, salad greens, oranges, grapefruits, and pineapple. Quite similarly, chewy food textures can be found in a variety of shellfish items including shrimp, scallops, and sushi. Consuming these foods will require consistent monitoring of intake habits. Optimal eating mechanics will need to be applied at all times in order to foster positive tolerance. Eating mechanics may also include (aside from chewing thoroughly while eating very slowly) consuming foods individually and not in combination with any other food. Consuming a single food at a meal can certainly enhance overall tolerance of intake because only one specific texture exists at that given time. Eating two or more different foods at a meal changes the style of chewing because foods present with an array of various textures thus creating more difficulty in executing effective mastication techniques. It may also be discovered that changing the fiber content through different cooking strategies will promote better tolerance. These strategies entail over cooking or soaking the fiber content out of food so the texture is less dense.

Tough food texture can be found in a variety of meats including steak, pork, veal, white meat chicken, and turkey, as well as sausage. A certain degree of toughness can also develop in well-cooked egg whites (whether separated from the yolk or cooked together).

To improve the tolerance of tough textured foods try implementing the following suggestions:

    a. Let food soak in marinade before cooking.
    b. Cook with marinades, sauce, or gravy.
    c. Cook food in a pressure cooker, crock-pot, or a casserole dish.
    d. Cook food at a lower temperature for a longer period of time.
    e. Crumble a cracker into the whites of the egg while cooking.

Apart from foods that are of chewy-tough consistency, there are some foods that are consumed quite easily, however, once settling in the stomach pouch they "expand" in size. This occurrence is very typical with foods that re-hydrate when cooked, such as pasta and rice. Bread products also display a certain degree of size enhancement and may be difficult to tolerate once in the pouch due to the "sponge-like" effect of the dough. This is especially true with doughy bread products such as bagels, rolls, and Italian bread. Bread products that lend themselves to better tolerance are a reduced-calorie brand bread, wraps, pita, as well as, flat breads.

To improve the tolerance of all bread products, particularly breads of doughy consistency, try implementing the following suggestions:

    a. Toast all bread before consuming. Bread that has been toasted crumbles upon the first bite, which eliminates the sponge-like effect.
    b. Remove the inside of doughy bread and then toast the outer area before consuming. Discarding the extra dough within bread products such as bagels, rolls, and Italian bread also eliminates the sponge effect.

3. Will there be any social or lifestyle ramifications in living with the Lap-Band?

One of the primary goals of Lap-Band intervention is for the opportunity to integrate surgical techniques within a variety of individual lifestyles. Key behavioral strategies have been found to improve the effectiveness of surgery, however, in many cases, habitual changes in lifestyle must occur in order for success to be achieved. Struggles in changing habits to effectively implement the Lap-Band are anticipated; however, as people learn to adapt to post-banded life, positive behaviors will become less tedious, and over time, can begin to feel more like second nature.

Surgical intervention is not intended to be implemented as a "diet," but rather to encourage (D)eveloping (I)deal (E)ating (T)echniques. Dieting implies instituting temporary changes to particular areas of food consumption. Recommendations after surgery are not given to avoid or eliminate certain foods (e.g., the no carbohydrate diet). Comparatively, recommendations to eat only certain foods (e.g., protein only) are also not provided. Adherence to a specific diet is not suggested, as dieting seems to be strongly correlated with feelings of deprivation. Not being permitted to eat in accordance with innate physiological and psychological desires will eventually conjure up feelings of deprivation. Deprivation of intake could then possibly lead to a loss of control in relationship to how, what, and when food should be consumed.

Dieting is intended to place control on an external entity. This entity can be a variety of externally directed tactics including menus, food plans, lists of appropriate foods, or suggestions for replacement meals. Through the help of Lap-Band surgery, external factors become less important while internal control becomes more valuable. Furthermore, when internal control is executed from a place of undeniable physical awareness, ideal eating techniques become more easily executed.

These techniques should focus on meeting a person's lifestyle and commitment to engaging in the most favorable behaviors that will enhance total well being. Ideal eating techniques need to be applied even more specifically to an individual's social circle. Social circles can be as close as everyday family members, co-workers, or people in association with at gatherings such as parties, weddings, vacations, and other celebrations.

Attending gatherings after surgical intervention can be socially challenging for some people. The challenge lies most often in the decision whether or not to disclose the fact that surgical treatment has taken place. Sharing information related to your band endeavor is, without question, a personal choice. Most recipients of the Lap-Band have little apprehension as to who knows of their surgical procedure. They may feel a deep-seated level of comfort, making it natural to share their surgical "story" with everyone regardless if one inquires, or not.

Some individuals are more selective in discussing their treatment with others. These individuals may choose only to discuss surgery with those individuals that are of close relation (spouse, partner, children, or other family members). This decision may be made based on the belief that their efforts of managing their weight through the assistance of surgical intervention will be supported by those they love. There may also be the understanding that eating habits amongst those who are of close relation will be affected, for the most part in a positive manner.

A small sector of individuals choose only to inform those in their lives who must know for personal reasons. These reasons may occur out of medical, financial, or emotional need. An even fewer number of people decide to keep their undertaking of the Lap-Band procedure solely between themselves and the medical-surgical team of practitioners. Beyond the community of physicians who can provide long-term care, some individuals may never desire or want to disclose their weight loss intervention.

Regardless of how an individual feels about revealing their undertaking of this surgical procedure, invitations to social gatherings will still exist. As with any other socially involved situation, three types of people will cross your path—those who are supportive, those who are not supportive, and those who simply leave you alone.

The majority of people who have witnessed your weight struggles will understandingly support your decision to undergo surgical weight loss intervention. There may be others whom for whatever reason are not supportive of your treatment endeavor. Their inability to support your pursuit may stem from a variety of reasons.

Jealousy is one of the main reasons underlying non-supportive behavior. All forms of jealousy exist out of fear. Feelings of fear by another individual may develop from insecurity. Insecurity with oneself, or specifically with personal weight issues, may be the underlying cause of fear and jealousy. Not being able to successfully treat one's weight condition, whether through traditional measures or as a potential surgical candidate, could limit the person's capacity to show support of another, despite the level of closeness.

The key aspect to social acceptance begins with you. Finding a level of comfort within you will make any situation more positive. Developing a foundation of confidence through self-discovery can help in dealing with the way others treat you. Paramount to social adaptation is surrounding by people who exhibit holistic well being- healthy body, mind, and spirit.

Supportive Services

An important but often overlooked benefit in meeting with a registered dietitian and psychologist for a mandatory pre-operative evaluation is to become enlightened on the fact that Lap-Band intervention is just the first step on a journey towards empowered wellness. A journey that has led to many previous unsuccessful outcomes can now be reversed through effective implementation of the Lap-Band's unique features.

The concept can be likened to venturing out into a snowstorm with either a four-wheel drive or a jalopy that has very poor traction in dangerous driving conditions. Both automobiles could provide safe and efficient transportation, however it is not difficult to foresee that the four-wheel drive possesses better driving capabilities to ensure that you will reach your destination safely and with the least amount of trouble. This situation is akin to utilizing the Lap-Band in place of non-surgical weight loss programs.

Non-surgical obesity treatment is bound to fail for most obese individuals because like the jalopy, these treatment modalities do not possess the proven entities for successful weight loss to occur. The underlying factor governing weight loss is consuming fewer calories than metabolically needed. The Lap-Band is designed to assist with caloric modification by virtue of two main properties:

1. Physical restriction - Constricting the stomach upon placement of the band creates a "virtual" pouch, which in all actuality is simply the top of the stomach that now lies above the band. To assist in visualizing this anatomical configuration, think of placing a belt around your waist. When wearing a belt, the stomach sits in different aliment with the lower body. Your stomach could feel tucked in closer to the body or it may lie over the belt. All body parts are still as one; however, the belt now separates the upper and lower body regions, similar to placing the band on the stomach. Lap-Band placement creates an upper and lower stomach region that is still in conjunction with both halves, however, both areas are not as "free to flow." The inability of food to pass as easily from the pouch to the stomach helps to create and sustain fullness. Although feelings of fullness do not necessarily negate continued consumption when normal physiology exists, it will be nearly impossible to continue eating with the band once physical fullness is achieved. Assimilation of food in a small reservoir (the upper stomach pouch) will ultimately limit the intake of additional food (and subsequently fewer calories).
2. Feeling satiated - Simple placement of the Lap-Band beneficially reduces fluctuations in appetite and subsequent hunger. This phenomenon, although not yet fully understood in bariatric medicine, is believed to be associated with the stimulation

of certain hormones and nerves that function as regulators of appetite. With a given quantity of food consumption, the stomach pouch will appropriately distend and nerves governing brain-satiation will be stimulated.

Aside from the physical aspects of surgery, support may be needed in the form of individual therapy, group meetings or even through contacts via the Internet or phone. The type of support received should be governed not only as it relates to feasibility, but also based on individual comfort. Some people may only desire to discuss certain issues with a therapist or counselor. Individual therapy is a safe environment for people to explore personal barriers to achieving successful weight loss. Others may feel less inhibited and more connected through participating in group therapy sessions. A skilled practitioner must mediate support meetings; otherwise, effective group interaction could be inhibited by disruptive and non-cohesive behavior.

Most insurance companies (and therefore many bariatric medical practices) require attending at least one support group before undergoing surgery. It is now common practice for surgical teams (consisting of a physician, physician assistant, psychologist, and nutritionist) to host interactive educational meetings where both pre and post-surgical patients can share ideas and knowledge or simply ask questions. It is also an inviting forum for people to express concerns regarding surgery or the challenges they have, or foresee having, with regards to instituting necessary lifestyle changes. Benefits of these meetings include preparing individuals for surgery, as well as assisting others on their quest for optimal weight management.

In addition to information-oriented meetings, supportive therapy can also be provided within discussion groups that are topic specific and contain fewer attendants. A psychologist and/or nutritionist often oversee these groups, as their expertise can be of valuable assistance. Maintaining the number of group participants within a range of fifteen to twenty (compared to a hundred or more attendants at general education-orientated meetings) will help manage an individually tailored therapy session. If individual or group sessions are not where someone desires to seek support, a non-confrontational option can be made through communication over the Internet or by phone.

There are weight loss practices that perform bariatric surgery, but do not have either the means or desire to assist with follow-up care. In addition, some individuals have had a poor outcome with surgical intervention and, therefore, cannot objectively provide support to others. Regardless of where you may gain support, it is important to be certain that you are seeking help from a reputable source, or in the case of a post-surgical patient, be certain that the individual has your best interest at heart.

Tips for Dining Out

1. Try ordering a balanced meal in an appetizer size portion.

Not only could this option potentially save you money, but it may also enable you to make food choices based on content rather than serving size.
If this option is not available, then consider

a) Sharing a meal
b) Bringing leftovers home

2. Choose foods based on familiar tolerance.

Always try food at home first before consuming that 'specific' food when dining out. Many people develop an anxiety-driven intolerance when trying certain foods for the very first time. Consuming foods you have tolerated well within the comforts of your home initially could help to prevent any intolerance due to feelings of anxiety and/or nervousness.

3. Order a meal that contains solid to semi-solid protein and vegetables.

To obtain adequate and prolonged satiation, banded patients are encouraged to consume a diet rich in solid to semi-solid consistency protein-based foods and vegetables. These two foods have been shown to effectively distend the pouch so the nerves of satiety can be stimulated in a long-lasting manner. If however there is a certain level of anxiety associated at that particular dining experience, it may be beneficial to consume a small quantity of softer consistency foods at the beginning of the meal followed by foods that are solid and digest slower.

4. Order water or any other non-carbonated, calorie free beverage.

Carbonation and calories are not something you want from liquids post-surgery. Carbonation is not well tolerated due to the gas release within the small stomach pouch. Calories consumed in the form of liquids will not benefit the effects of post-surgery satiation. Remember to drink your beverage of choice before the meal, not with or for approximately one hour following your intake. If needed, take small sips of your beverage at the meal or shortly thereafter, however the less you drink the better. This will help sustain optimal full-ness and prevent any tendency of intolerance due to over filling your stomach pouch.

5. Have your meal cooked in a way that will optimize tolerance.

You will come to realize that certain foods need to be prepared in a specific way in order to ensure an uneventful intake. This may mean adding gravy and sauce to soften foods. Especially with protein foods, cooking at less temperature for a lower duration will prevent an end product that is too dry, tough, or chewy.

6. Portion food on smaller plate.

Ask for smaller, dessert-type plates to portion the quantity of food you are intending to consume. Then ask for the remainder of your meal to be immediately wrapped in a "to go" container. This will help prevent over eating based on what your eyes are seeing. Remember you always want to eat based on internal awareness, not external cues.

7. Spend time cutting all food into baby size bites (the size of an eraser) before the start of the meal.

By cutting all food in this manner before taking the first bite, you significantly reduce the likelihood of intolerance caused by a blockage at the band-pouch junction. Less time and effort will be required to break down baby size bites compared to the size an adult would take.

8. Consume protein and vegetable before the start of a carbohydrate source.

Eating protein and vegetable foods in their entirety will ensure the positive effects of sa-tiation. If tolerated, consume a smaller portion of carbohydrate rich foods towards the end of the meal for satisfying intake along with bringing the meal into nutritional balance.

9. Pay close attention to the amount of time it takes to complete your meal.

Although you are encouraged to take twenty minutes to consume a meal, taking longer can lessen feelings of satiation. As you eat, some of the food passes through the upper stomach pouch leaving room for additional food. Therefore, by taking an extended period of time at your meal, you can ultimately consume more food than in a shorter time frame.

Taking up to an hour or longer to consume a meal is in essence "grazing". Grazing is a habit associated with consuming small amounts of food during shorter spaced intervals. Engaging in this habit while living with the band will not allow you to gain the most benefit from your surgical tool because it negates the effect of filling and distending the pouch all at one interval to maximize satiation.

10. As always, devote full focused attention to ensure adequate chewing.

Failure to commit to chewing food to a mushy consistency can lead to painful discomfort. If the discomfort is extreme it can further induce the need to vomit and/or regurgitation. If this were to occur, it is important to switch to a liquid meal rather than the meal at hand. Liquids will safely flow through the pouch, which can be swollen and irritated because of the prior degree of food intolerance.

Soft-Calorie Syndrome

Comfort foods are defined as those foods we rely on to induce relaxation, ease stress, and are often ones that evoke positive memories. Whether or not the statement "Food Equals Love" is true, food has become a symbolic representation of nurturing. After all, wellness is not just about good nutrition, but it also includes developing enriching relationships in which an exchange of healthy emotions can be shared. Enduring relations with others while sustaining a balanced emotional state is an important aspect toward living a life of balance and wholeness. When food consumption is abused to a level of compulsive overeating, relationships and personal emotions can suffer.

In the field of bariatrics, soft-calorie syndrome has been designated to reflect the intake of calorie-rich foods, which contain a large percent of fat and sugar. These foods can be tempting, because either they represent a sense of comfort or because nutrient dense foods like lean protein, vegetables, fruits, and whole grains are not highly desired due to the requirement of slower consumption, extensive chewing and a greater degree of patience. Soft-calorie foods will dissolve very easily with minimal chewing effort, thereby passing through the pouch quickly. This means that a larger volume of soft-calorie foods can be consumed at one time with very limited satiation. Weight loss can thus be hindered, or even more concerning, weight gain can be experienced.

Soft-calorie syndrome appears to affect patients who have a significant level of restriction within the Lap-Band. This may be the case, as it becomes more challenging to tolerate solid consistency foods because of the extensive chewing requirement. If this is the reason, patients are encouraged to discuss their situation with a medical team member. It may then be decided, collaboratively, that a reduction in saline would promote optimal tolerance of nutrient-dense, solid foods—

The Ultimate Goal for Lap-Band Recipients!!!

Do not become trapped in the soft-calorie syndrome. Seek advice on adjusting the level of restriction with your band to allow for the intake of nutrient dense food at an appropriate quantity without possibly compromising health and weight loss by eating non-nutritious, soft-calorie foods.

In addition, if you discover that you are consuming soft, high-calorie foods from a place of emotional need, then you must work toward resolving this need through establishing effective behavioral strategies, either individually or with the help of another, such as a therapist.

First Bite Syndrome

"First Bite Syndrome" relates to the inability for continued food consumption after taking the initial bite. Inability of consumption is indicative of an obstruction in the banded-pouch area. This obstruction or blockage is primarily the result of consuming a bite size that is too large for the opening between the band and the remaining stomach. Consequently, pain and discomfort will occur until the situation is resolved. More than likely, pressure radiating from the pouch to the esophagus will induce regurgitation of food up through the mouth.

If and when this occurs, it is best to first try and relax so that any form of emotional distress can be controlled in the best possible manner. Next, take a mental recap of the given situation and make a written notation of the behaviors that lead up to this episode. Proceed by answering the following questions.

- Did I take a very small bite of food?
- How well did I chew the food before swallowing?
- Was I distracted in any way from focusing on appropriately executing necessary intake behaviors?

After evaluating the incident, develop a strategic plan that will help prevent another episode of the first bite syndrome. Some strategies may include cutting all food to be consumed in very small pieces (the size of an eraser at the end of a pencil) before beginning a meal. By consuming one small piece at a time, the first bite syndrome can be avoided. On a final note, liquids should only be consumed for the remainder of the meal to dissolve any irritation that may have occurred due to regurgitation. Liquids or soft, mushy foods should only then be consumed at the next meal to help optimize continued tolerance.

Intolerance to food can occur at any point at the meal—beginning, middle, and/or end. When intolerance occurs at some point during the meal (middle to end), more than likely the inability to consume the food is related to over consumption of food within the pouch. When this occurs, the pouch is unable to distend maximally to accompany the extra food that has been consumed. Strategizing to improve portion control would be of tremendous benefit in this given situation because the intolerance was related to over consumption and not necessarily inadequate chewing.

Vitamin-Mineral Supplementation Following Lap-Band Surgery

Vitamin-mineral deficiencies can develop in patients who have a purely restrictive operation such as the Lap-Band. These deficiencies may develop secondary to

1. excessive regurgitation or vomiting of food and/or
2. consumption of a soft-calorie diet due to intolerance's and avoidance of more nutritious foods such as meat, vegetables, and fruits.

To prevent vitamin-mineral deficiencies from occurring, it is essential that all Lap-Band recipients supplement their diet with a multivitamin-mineral daily. Additional vitamins can always be consumed as advised by a physician or taken based upon an individual's health needs.

Due to the restrictive nature of surgery, many patients have a better tolerance to chewable, liquid, or powdered vitamins. Patient's can decide to take either

1. two children's chewable multivitamin's daily (e.g., Flintstone's Complete),
2. one adult chewable multivitamin daily (e.g., Centrum), or
3. the equivalent of one adult multivitamin in liquid form daily (e.g., Centrum).

Keep in mind however, that following surgery, your body may not efficiently metabolize standard vitamins because most commercial vitamins contain fillers, binders, and coatings. These byproducts counteract with dilution, resulting in a low concentration of nutrients. Therefore, you may want to consider purchasing multivitamin and mineral formulas that have been specifically engineered to meet the needs of bariatric surgical patients.

If you are serious about adding an optimal bariatric vitamin formula to your diet, then you must consider the information provided on the following page (64).

The Trump Network's revolutionary Priva Test eliminates the guesswork and confusion from personal supplementation. The simple in-home test scientifically answers what vitamins, minerals and vital nutrients your individual body needs every day.

Developed in partnership with one of the world's foremost nutritional laboratories, The Trump Network has a team of experts analyzing your specific metabolic markers from the in-home Priva Test. This process has eliminated the obsolete one-size fits all vitamin mentality and scientific high-technology solutions to each individual seeking optimal health.

Your Priva Test will determine the scientific nutritional design for your Custom Essentials daily formula. Following an analysis of laboratory results, your Personal Custom Essentials formula will provide your body with 50 pharmaceutical-grade nutrients in a whole food base combining- Antioxidants, Chelated Minerals, Phytonutrients and Whole vitamin Complexes.

For less than $2.00 a day, you can obtain your Personal Custom Essential formula to help optimize your health and well-being. Each 30-day supply of your Custom Essential formula is individually wrapped for convenient-daily use.

Not only are Custom Essentials specifically formulated to meet your individual nutritional needs, but also they are extremely east to consume through a restricted bariatric weight loss tool such as gastric banding or bypass. Do not miss out on supplementing your dietary regimen with these innovative vitamins-minerals.

Order today at: www.trumpnetwork.com/lisamariegentile

Before pursuing surgical weight loss intervention, it is important to take a positive look on what it truly means to D.I.E.T.

D eveloping

I deal

E ating

T echniques

These techniques should reflect your commitment to engaging in the most favorable behaviors that will enhance your lifestyle and total well-being!

Recommended Pre-Operative Nutrition Plan

In preparation for surgery, patients are instructed to stop their normal dietary consumption one week (7 days)* before surgery and replace their intake with a recommended "Modified Liquid Meal Plan."

*The recommended 7 day time period may be adjusted to include more (10-14) or less (4-5) time depending on weight status and stomach girth. Recommendations should be individualized by each patient's bariatric physician and/or nutritionist.

A modified liquid meal plan, reduced in both calories and fat, will provide a number of benefits including:

1. *Reducing the size of the liver, thus improving exposure to the surgical area.*
   The liver can become infiltrated with dense fatty tissue as weight accumulates, as well as when the diet is rich in fat and calories. At the time of surgery, the liver is retracted due to its close proximity to the surgical site. If the liver is too dense (fatty) and cannot be proficiently retracted, the surgery may be too difficult to perform.

2. *Promotion of beneficial weight loss.*
   Depending on pre-operative weight status, gender, and adherence to the pre-operative modified liquid meal plan, pre-surgical patients can lose approximately 2 to 4 percent of weight.

3. *Psychological adaptation to post-operative requirements.*
   Although the pre-operative modified liquid meal plan can be more challenging than the recommended liquid plan following surgery, patients gain valuable awareness as it relates to the consumption of appropriate protein enriched beverages along with instituting effective intake habits. Ultimately, transition to early post-banded life is much easier.

The pre-operative modified liquid meal plan is designed to provide moderate caloric intake consumed over the course of **six daily meals.** Consuming multiple meals of equal caloric content, evenly distributed throughout the day helps improve adherence while limiting fluctuations in both one's appetite and food cravings.

Although the pre-operative modified liquid meal plan is structured to provide a consistent intake of approximately **200 calories per meal (1200 daily calories)** that are enriched in protein, modified in carbohydrate, and low in fat; it can be *customized* to meet a patient's *nutritional* and *medical needs* as well as *individual preferences* and/or *tolerances*.

Recommended Pre-Operative Nutrition Plan

Those suffering with **diabetes** before surgery are strongly encouraged to discuss the recommended pre-operative modified liquid meal plan with their doctor so medication can be adjusted appropriately. Immediately post-surgery, modification in medication will be tailored to meet individual needs by the bariatric physician. Following that point, changes in medication would be monitored by a personal physician.

Keep in mind making a commitment to modify your daily consumption and habits of intake before surgery will help ensure a good surgical outcome along with enhancing your adjustment to life after surgery. If there is a special occasion that occurs during the time period when the recommended pre-operative modified liquid meal is advised, and you decide to eat food in place of a liquid meal; remember to make sensible choice. Limit the intake of high fat foods, pay close attention to portion control, and get back on track as soon as the occasion has ended.

The Pre-operative Modified Liquid Meal Plan consists of...

Full Liquids for Six Consecutive days (Days 1 - 6).

Followed by...

Clear Liquids on the Last day, (Day 7) - one day prior to surgery.

Surgery would be scheduled to occur on the Eighth day.*
*The time period may be adjusted depending on multiple factors including body weight. Abide by what has been individually recommended to you by your physician and/or nutritionist.

Full Liquids are of cloudy consistency and contain beneficial protein, however these liquid items also contain various levels of fat; therefore non-fat and/or low-fat items (1 to 3 grams of fat per serving) are recommended.

Full Liquids include: **Milk** (with or without additional noted ingredients), **Pudding, Yogurt, Soup,** as well as, **Recommended Meal Replacement Beverages**.

Clear Liquids are of a transparent consistency and contain limited calories and thus insignificant protein, carbohydrate, and fat content.

Clear Liquids include: **Jell-O Gelatin** (any color)**, Flavored Ice** (any color)**, Broth, Tea,** and **Clear Fruit Juice** (without pulp such as Apple Juice and/or White Grape Juice).

Recommended Pre-Operative Nutrition Plan

Before providing detailed information pertaining to the pre-operative modified liquid plan, the following information discusses the importance of ... Meal Replacement Beverages.

Meal Replacement Beverages

Meal Replacement Beverages are scientifically formulated liquids that provide the body with a balance of nutrients that contain "a greater concentration of protein for every calorie."

Meal replacement beverages are notably beneficial during the pre-operative modified full liquid phase because of their unique nutritional content, however, meal replacement beverages are *not of extreme importance until after surgery*.

The main reason meal replacement beverages are not of significance until after surgery lies in the fact that the quantity of liquids consumed before surgery is at an adequate (yet significantly reduced) level, thus providing sufficient protein. Adequate nourishment pre-operatively can be obtained from traditional full liquids such as non-fat milk, pudding and yogurt as well as low-fat soups.

Following surgery, fewer calories of enriched protein content is needed to ensure optimal, safe weight loss while allowing for complete healing of the skin and muscle tissue. Therefore, meal replacement beverages are of *significant importance during the post-operative full liquid plan*.

Although various meal replacement beverages are available for purchase at many health food and vitamin stores, there is no standard regulation as to the "true" ingredients contained in these beverages. Ingredients listed on the nutritional label may in fact not be accurate due to the lack of FDA testing.

Medifast is one of the most recommended medical-based meal replacement beverages. **Medifast** products can be purchased by following the information on page 70-71.

Regardless of which meal replacement beverage you choose, it is important to purchase these beverages before surgery. This will ensure that the beverage is readily available for your consumption once arriving home from the hospital.

Recommended Pre-Operative Nutrition Plan

If purchasing meal replacement beverages from a health food or vitamin store, and not Medifast, look for a product that contains…

- **Approximately 100 calories** (+ or - 10 to 20 calories) in **8-ounces** with
  - *Greater than* **12 grams Protein**
  - *Less than* **3 grams Fat** and
  - ***Between* 8** and **13 grams Carbohydrate-** dependent upon protein & fat content.

If consuming a meal replacement beverage ***pre-operatively***, you may drink up to **16 ounces** per meal for a total of *200 calories*.

When consuming a meal replacement beverage ***post-operatively,*** reduce the intake to **8 ounces** per meal for a total of *100 calories*.

Pay attention when purchasing ***powdered meal replacement beverages*** because these beverages are typically recommended for preparation with juice or milk. The calories contained in an 8-ounce serving of juice or non-fat milk are however equal to the total number of calories recommended for the entire post-operative meal (100 calories). Therefore, mixing the powdered meal replacement beverage with 8 oz. of juice or non-fat milk will double the total calories, thus, exceeding your daily needs post-operative.

Mixing the powdered meal replacement beverage with water is the best option, however, if flavor and/or consistency cannot be tolerated, then alternative options includes mixing the powdered meal replacement with

- 4 oz. of water and 4 oz. of non-fat milk or
- 4 oz. of water and 4 oz. of fruit (apple) juice.

Both options will help reduce the number of calories consumed per meal while providing optimal protein consumption.

Recommended Pre-Operative Nutrition Plan

MEDIFAST is a medically prescribed liquid meal replacement that will provide you with one of the best formulas for protein, vitamins, and beneficial macronutrient intake.

When considering which Medifast product to purchase, keep in mind that all listed beverages contain the same content. It does not matter which products you choose. Choices are made individually based on preference of flavor and convenience of intake.

Medifast- Ready to Drink Formula (RTD) does not require mixing:

1. **RTD Shakes** – flavors include chocolate and vanilla.

Medifast- Powdered Formulas that need to be mixed with water include:

2. **Medifast – 55 Shake** – flavors include choc, van, straw, orange, banana, and mocha.

3. **Medifast Plus Appetite Suppression Shakes** – flavors include choc. and vanilla.

4. **Iced Tea** (peach and raspberry) **and Fruit Drinks** – non-dairy.

5. **Chai-Latte, Cappuccino, and Hot Cocoa-** Great tasting hot beverages.

6. **Antioxidant Shake-** flavors include blueberry, cherry pomegranate, and dark chocolate.

Recommended Pre-Operative Nutrition Plan

To Purchase Medifast Liquid Meal Replacements Visit:

www.LisaGentile.tsfl.com
Or Call:
1-800-572-4417

When calling in an order, be sure to state that you are a new customer. You will then be asked to provide a Health Advisor I.D. # 3670401

How Much to Order:

Patients will need an estimated total of ~ 85 – 95 Liquid Meal Replacements.
These beverages are divided as follows:
Pre-surgical intake ~ 12-24 (~2 – 4 daily for 6 days, depending upon individual preference)
Post-surgical intake during **Full Liquid Plan 56** (4 daily for 14 days)
Post-surgical intake during **Soft Food Plan** ~14 (1 daily for 14 days)

Recommended Pre-Operative Nutrition Plan

Full Liquids to choose from during Days 1- 6 include:

1. **Skim, Skim Plus, 1%, Soy, or Non/Low-fat Organic Milk**–meal serving= **8 oz.**
   To enhance flavor and consistency of milk, you can blend 8 ounces of milk with ice and either **Carnation Instant Breakfast Beverage** (No-added sugar) or **Alba mix**. This milk beverage mixture can also include a small quantity of **fresh or frozen fruit** (e.g., handful of berries, ¼ banana) for additional flavor.

2. **Pudding** – *Non-fat* and *No-added sugar* – meal serving size = **12 oz.**
   (**'Jell-O Brand'** Sugar-Free, Fat Free (boxed item-follow directions for preparation on the package; prepare with Skim, Skim-Plus, 1%, Soy, or non/low-fat Organic Milk). Many ready-to-eat puddings are fat-free **or** sugar-free and *not both* (fat-free **and** sugar-free). If ready-to-eat pudding is desired, it is better to purchase **Fat-Free** pudding *with sugar* rather than Sugar-Free pudding with fat.

3. **Yogurt** – *Non-fat* and *No-added sugar* – meal serving size = **12 oz.**
   (**Axelrod, Columbo-Light, Dannon-Light, Stoneyfield** (organic), **Turkey Hill** (frozen)) Yogurt can be frozen and fruit flavored as well.

4. **Fage** and/or **Chobani Greek Yogurt** - *Total 0% Fat* – meal serving size = **8 oz.**
   Mixed with 6 oz. of **fresh** or **canned fruit** (100% juice content) - such as 1/2 banana, 3/4 cup strawberries or 3/4 cup canned pears.

5. **Soups** – *Low-fat* **(3 or less grams of fat per serving)** – meal serving size = **16 - 20 oz.**
   (**Healthy Choice, Pritikin, and Healthy Valley** are soups that are low in fat & sodium) *"Chunky Consistency Soups,"* containing ingredients such as chicken, turkey, noodles, rice, and vegetables can be consumed pre-operative; however, for a short time following surgery, modifications must be made to the chunky consistency for promotion of optimal tolerance. *Homemade soup* is a great alternative to canned soup; remember to keep the fat content to a minimal level. *Avoid eating all creamed soups*, unless they are low in fat. In addition, **consume no more than two soup meals per day** because of the sodium and chunky food content.

6. **Medifast Liquid Meal Replacements**, (along with other appropriate protein-enriched meal replacements, as discussed on pages 68-71) – meal serving size = 16 oz.

Recommended Pre-Operative Nutrition Plan

Clear Liquids to choose from on Day 7 (one day prior to surgery) **include:**

- **Broth, Jell-O, Ice, Clear Fruit Juice,** and **Tea.**
  - All clear liquids (unless otherwise specified by your physician) should be **regular** and *(not sugar-free)* for obtainment of beneficial calories.
  - Vary your quantity of clear liquids based on your appetite, thirst, and energy level.

Recommended Pre-Operative Nutrition Plan

Behavior Strategies to help during the Pre-Operative Liquid Phase include:

1. Consume **6 liquid meals** daily.

   Menus are provided to assist with meal planning, however you can always vary choices based upon individual preference and/or tolerance. Be certain though to make appropriate substitutions.

   If your appetite is insatiable, you can consume one additional liquid meal per day as needed. On the contrary, if your appetite is well controlled while consuming less than six meals per day, then that is acceptable as well.

   Meals can be consumed in any order or combination, including consuming two different liquids at the same meal. If this is desired, liquids must be reduced to an appropriate quantity. For example, instead of consuming 12 oz. of either pudding or yogurt at one meal, you may decide to consume 6 oz. of pudding and 6 oz. of yogurt at the same meal for a total of 12 oz.

   In addition, if it is too difficult to schedule six meals daily, then one or two meals can contain double the quantity. This will provide a plan of four to five meals daily, but with the same number of calories. Be aware however that for a short-time following surgery, six daily meals is highly recommended for a number of reasons including assuring adequate nutrition while consuming substantially reduced portions and limited calories. Inability to consume adequate quantity occurs initially due to tissue swelling (edema), which is a normal side effect from Lap-Band surgical implantation. In turn, meal servings are significantly reduced to ensure that adequate healing of the stomach pouch occurs without causing undue pressure. Unnecessary pressure to the newly placed band can lead to complications of placement.

   Adapting to a **six-meal-a-day schedule one week prior to surgery** can help transition to the same schedule when most needed during the **two-week post-operative full liquid plan.**

2. With the intake of multiple lactose products, you may experience **cramps, bloating, gas and/or diarrhea while consuming full liquids**. If this occurs, try taking Lactaid Ease Chewable products, Dairy Care, or switch to Lactaid, Dairy Ease, Soy, or Almond Milk to ease the intolerance.

3. Consume a **liquid meal ~ every 2 to 3 hours** to prevent excessive hunger.

   Consistent intake while adhering to a low (1200) calorie liquid plan will help stabilize blood sugar so energy levels and appetite do not become unmanageable. Waiting too long between meals can cause blood sugar levels to drop very low. A severe drop in blood sugar can then lead to a desire for calories and/or foods that are not recommended.

4. Consume **unlimited water** (at least 64 oz.) or any flavored, non-caloric water beverages (e.g., crystal-lite, diet iced tea, etc.) throughout the day.

Recommended Pre-Operative Nutrition Plan

5. **Diet-carbonated** beverages can be consumed pre-operatively, however, these beverages are not recommended after surgery due to poor tolerance and the belief that excessive intake over time can disrupt the structural integrity of the stomach pouch.

6. **Fruit juice** beverages should be restricted to no more than 6 oz. per day to assist with calorie control. **Vegetable juice** beverages can be consumed in moderation of 12 oz. daily.

7. **Coffee** and **tea** can continue to be consumed in moderation, however remember to rehydrate by consuming 16 oz. of water for every 8 oz. of caffeine containing coffee or tea beverage.

8. If needed, **diet Jell-O**, **broth,** and/or **no-added sugar ices** can be consumed in moderation along with your six full liquid meals during days one to six to help satisfy cravings.

   Pudding and Yogurt have natural lactose (milk) sugar and are not *Sugar-Free*. When buying no-added sugar yogurt and pudding, sugar substitutes (such as Nutra-Sweet (Aspartame) or Splenda) are typically added to provide a sweeter taste without additional calories. Organic substitutions are a much healthier option. Organic products are made from natural milled cane sugar rather than artificial sugar sweeteners. Sugar substitutes have been discovered to contain unnatural ingredients that can potentially cause the body to develop disease.

9. **Typically the first three days** of the **pre-operative** nutrition plan are the most challenging, both physically and psychologically, due to a transition from regular foods to full liquids. The difficulty may lie not only from consuming fewer calories, but also due to the **absence of chewing**.

   To assist in this transition you can consume the following items…in *addition* to your six full-liquid meals.

   1. **Crackers** (10 to 15 plain, saltine type)
   2. **Fresh Fruit** (1 to 2 medium size or one cup of cut-up fruit)
   3. **Raw, Steamed or Grilled Vegetables** (1 to 2 cups)

   All three items (Crackers, Fruits, and Vegetables)* can be consumed in the quantity provided during Days one to three, however the…*less you eat, the better*.
   *It is best to avoid eating crackers, fruits, and vegetables after day three of the seven-day plan. If struggles present, continued intake is acceptable, but not on day 7-Clear Liquids only.
   If desired, fat-free salad dressing or spray butter can be added to vegetables or crackers. Avoid eating peas and corn. Salad ingredients such as croutons, nuts, seeds, olives, etc. are also not recommended.

Sample Pre-operative Liquid Menu

	Day #1	Day #2	Day #3	Day #4	Day #5	Day #6	Day #7
Meal #1	12 oz. Yogurt– Non-fat, No-added sugar	16 oz. = 2 (8 oz.) Liquid Meal Replacement- Medifast	12 oz. Pudding- Non-fat, No-added Sugar	16 oz. = 2 (8 oz.) Liquid Meal Replacement- Medifast	8 oz. Skim Milk mixed with ½ scoop Alba Mix Ice, as desired	12 oz. Pudding- Non-fat, No-added sugar	Jell-O- Unlimited
Meal #2	16 oz. = 2 (8 - oz.) Liquid Meal Replacement- Medifast	8 oz. Skim Milk mixed with ½ scoop Alba Mix Ice, as desired	16 oz. = 2 (8 oz.) Liquid Meal Replacement- Medifast	16 oz. Chicken Vegetable Soup- Low-fat	16 oz. = 2 (8 oz.) Liquid Meal Replacement- Medifast	8 oz. Skim Milk blended with handful of Blackberries	Apple Juice- Unlimited
Meal #3	16 oz. Turkey Vegetable Soup- Low-fat	16 oz. Chicken Noodle Soup- Low-fat	16 oz. Manhattan Clam Chowder Soup – Low-fat	8 oz. Fage Yogurt- mixed well with ¾ cup Blueberries	6 oz. Pudding- & 6 oz. Yogurt- Non-fat, No-added Sugar	16 oz. = 2 (8 oz.) Liquid Meal Replacement- Medifast	Broth- Unlimited
Meal #4	16 oz. = 2 (8 oz.) Liquid Meal Replacement- Medifast	8 oz. Fage Yogurt- Mixed well with ¾ cup canned Peaches	6 oz. Yogurt– & 6 oz. Pudding- Non-fat, No-added sugar	8 oz. Skim Milk blended with handful of Strawberries	16 oz. Turkey Rice Soup- Low-fat	6 oz. Pudding- & 6 oz. Yogurt- Non-fat, No-added sugar	Italian Ice- Unlimited
Meal #5	12 oz. Pudding- Non-fat, No-added sugar	20 oz. Egg Drop Soup	16 oz. Split Pea Soup- Low-fat	16 oz. Lentil Soup- Low-fat	12 oz. Frozen Yogurt- Non-fat, No added sugar	20 oz. Vegetable Beef Soup- Low-fat	Jell-O- Unlimited
Meal #6	8 oz. Skim Milk blended with ¼ Banana	12 oz. Pudding- Non-fat, No-added sugar	8 oz. Skim Milk mixed with (1) Carnation Bkfst Ice, as desired	12 oz. Pudding- Non-fat, No-added sugar	16 oz. = 2 (8 oz.) Liquid Meal Replacement- Medifast	12 oz. Pudding Non-fat, No-added sugar	White Grape Juice- Unlimited

Average Calories for each day = ~ 1200
Average grams of Carbohydrate each day = ~ 175

Average grams of Protein each day = ~ 85
Average grams of Fat each day = ~ 12

Recommended Post-Operative Nutrition Plan

While the tissue of your surgically altered stomach is healing, you should consume liquids and then progress to soft (mushy) foods before returning to a solid food plan. This modified consistency food plan will help prevent irritation at the surgery site and allow you to develop favorable eating habits.

Clear Liquids: Recommended for **1 day** following surgery.
Appropriate Clear Liquid items include the following:
Broth (low-sodium), Tea, Fruit Juice (Apple or White Grape), Jell-O Gelatin and Flavored Ice.

Full Liquids: Recommended for **2 weeks** following clear liquids – **Weeks 1 and 2.**
Appropriate Full Liquid items include the following:
Skim (+), 1% or Soy Milk, Carnation Instant Breakfast (no-added sugar), Alba mix, Soups (liquefied, low-fat, protein-based (i.e., cream of tomato)) & Non-fat, No-added sugar: Pudding and Yogurt.
Most importantly, Liquid Meal Replacements: such as Medifast.

Soft, Mushy Foods: Recommended for **2 weeks** following full liquids – **Weeks 3 and 4.** If desired, foods can be modified in a blender or a food processor until a semi-solid or mushy consistency is achieved. Fruit or vegetable juice, broth or skim milk may be mixed with the food to obtain desired consistency.
Appropriate Soft, Mushy Food items include the following:
soft boiled eggs, sliced thin (soft) cheese, cottage/ricotta cheese, tuna fish, egg/chicken/turkey salad, sliced thin luncheon meat, flaky fish, mashed meatball, grounded-minced dark chicken or turkey meat, beans, peanut butter (creamy), tofu, hot or cold-mushy cereal, skinless fruit, mashed potato, well-cooked (mushy) vegetables, saltine crackers, and chunky soups.

Solid Foods: **If no problems are experienced with soft-mushy foods, solid foods can then be started approximately 5 weeks after surgery.** Your long-term, optimal food plan consists of solid foods, which take both time and effort to consume slowly and chew thoroughly. Among solid foods, there are those foods, which are better tolerated and those that are more difficult. It may take time for you to optimally tolerate bread, pasta, rice, and red meat. To benefit from feelings of prolonged fullness, choose high quality food items at every meal, including finely cut-up lean protein (e.g., chicken, fish, turkey, or beef) with vegetables (raw, steamed, or grilled).

Recommended Post-Operative Nutrition Plan

While the tissues of your surgically altered stomach are healing, you will be on a variety of liquids for several weeks to prevent damage to your surgery site.

Clear Liquids are consumed on the first day following surgery.

BEHAVIOR STRATEGIES INCLUDE:

1. Consume **Clear Liquids** for **one full day** following surgery.
   Clear liquids will start in the hospital before going home the day after surgery.
   Continue drinking Clear Liquids until the morning of the second day post-operative.
   Full liquids are then recommended for two weeks.
2. **Plan** to consume **6 clear liquid meals daily**.
3. **Space** clear liquid **meals** approximately **2 to 3 hours apart**.
4. **Sip water** between all meals on a **constant basis**.
5. **Pace** meals so it takes **20 minutes** to consume a recommended **6 to 8 oz.** serving.
   Clear Liquids consist of:
   > Fruit Juice
   > Broth
   > Tea
   > Flavored Ice
   > Jell-O Gelatin

For a short time following surgery, sips of liquid will produce a feeling of desired fullness. **It is therefore, extremely important to consume clear liquids at a pace of…**

~ 1 ounce (size of medicine cup**) every two-three minutes.**

Straws with a large opening are not recommended because there is the possibility of overfilling your stomach pouch with liquid and air, which can cause pain and/or discomfort.
Carbonated beverages should be avoided at all times following surgery due to excessive gas formation with the possibility of stretching the pouch over time.

*Clear liquids can be consumed occasionally as your diet progresses, however, remember clear liquids lack beneficial calories and protein.

Recommended Post-Operative Nutrition Plan

Consume Full Liquids starting on the second day following surgery.

BEHAVIOR STRATEGIES INCLUDE:

1. Consume a **Full Liquid Plan** for **two weeks-** weeks 1 and 2 post-surgery.
2. **Plan** to consume **6**, nourishing **full liquid meals daily**.
3. **Space** full liquid **meals** approximately **2 to 3 hours apart**.
4. **Sip water** between all meals on a **constant basis**.

   Initially water intake should be at least 32 oz. and eventually (64 oz.) daily.
On account of only being able to consume small sips of water at one time, some individuals may experience difficulty meeting their hydration needs for a short-time following band placement. Try your best to consume at least half of the daily requirements (32 oz.). Over time, as water consumption becomes less tedious, 64 ounces will be easier to achieve on a daily basis.

   Although water is the preferred fluid of choice, all non-caloric, non-carbonated, decaffeinated beverages count toward your daily liquid consumption.

Please Note: Coffee or tea can also be consumed in moderation.

Water Intolerance: Some post-operative patients develop a funny taste in their mouth after consuming water and complain that ***water even tastes BAD***. This can lead to feelings of nausea and stomach cramping. To help improve water intake try
   (a) changing the water temperature—try ice cold and room temperature or
   (b) add flavor to the water with a splash of lemon (juice), orange, or sugar-free products such as crystal-lite, if desired.

5. **Pace** meals so it takes **10 minutes** to consume a recommended **6 to 8 oz. serving**. Sip liquids at a pace of approximately **2 oz. every two-three minutes.**
6. If purchasing an alternative beverage to Medifast, look for a product that contains 8 oz. in quantity with approximately 100 calories, greater than 12 grams protein, and less than 3 grams fat. Carbohydrate content will vary between 8 and 13 grams depending on protein and fat content.

Recommended Post-Operative Nutrition Plan

2 Week Full Liquid Plan Guidelines

Consume 4 Protein Enriched Liquid Meal Replacements Daily.

Recommended Liquid Meal Replacement: ***Medifast** - www.LisaGentile.tsfl.com or an *alternative, nutritionally appropriate product purchased from a health food store.*

To ensure adequate nutrient intake
consume 2 additional full liquid meals daily
from the list below:

- **Milk- Skim, Skim Plus, 1% or Soy** = 8 oz. serving
  Or
    - 6 oz. with **1/2 packet Carnation Instant Bkfst** (No-added sugar) + Ice- blend well.
    - 6 oz. with **1/2 scoop Alba mix** (Add ice and Blend well).
    - A small amount of fruit can also be blended with milk for added flavor.
- **Pudding-** *non-fat, no-added sugar* = 8 oz. (i.e., **Jell-O Brand** made with skim milk).
- **Yogurt-** *non-fat, no-added sugar* = 8 oz. (i.e., **Axelrod, Colombo-Light**, **Dannon-Light, Stoneyfield-organic (6 oz.) & Frozen Yogurt (Turkey Hill)**).
- **Fage** and/or **Chobani Greek Yogurt-** *Total 0% Fat-* meal serving = 6 oz. Yogurt can be blended with fresh or canned fruit.
- **Soups-***liquefied, low-fat:* **(3 or less grams of fat per serving)**
  Chunky Soups must be liquefied before consuming to prevent poor tolerance.
  Chunky Soups can be *liquefied* in either a *blender* or *food processor.*
  The final soup consistency should be able to consume through a straw.
    - Low-fat, Low-Sodium soup brands include:
        - **Healthy Choice, Pritikin, and Healthy Valley**
    - Examples of Appropriate Soup Choices include:
        - **Chicken/Turkey/Noodles/Rice/Vegetables** (liquefied) = 6 oz.
        - **Tomato soup** = 6 oz. (prepare with 6 oz. skim milk for extra protein)
        - **Cream potato soup** = 6 oz. (prepare with 6 oz. skim milk, stir well)
        - ***Split Pea** = 8 oz., ***Lentil** = 6 oz., ***Egg Drop** = 8 oz.

Please Note:
   *Soups of thicker consistency (such as split pea, lentil and egg drop) are safe to consume without modifying as long these soups are consumed at a very slow pace to ensure optimal tolerance.

Week 1 - Sample Post-operative Full Liquid Menu

	Day #1	Day #2	Day #3	Day #4	Day #5	Day #6	Day #7
Meal #1	(1) – 8 oz. Liquid Meal Replacement- Medifast	(1) – 8 oz. Liquid Meal Replacement- Medifast	6 oz. Skim Milk Mixed with ½ scoop Alba Ice, as desired	(1) – 8 oz. Liquid Meal Replacement- Medifast	(1) – 8 oz. Liquid Meal Replacement- Medifast	4 oz. Pudding- & 4 oz. Yogurt- Non-fat, No-added sugar	(1) – 8 oz. Liquid Meal Replacement- Medifast
Meal #2	(1) – 8 oz. Liquid Meal Replacement- Medifast	(1) – 8 oz. Liquid Meal Replacement- Medifast	(1) – 8 oz. Liquid Meal Replacement- Medifast	(1) – 8 oz. Liquid Meal Replacement- Medifast	(1) – 8 oz. Liquid Meal Replacement- Medifast	(1) – 8 oz. Liquid Meal Replacement- Medifast	(1) – 8 oz. Liquid Meal Replacement- Medifast
Meal #3	4 oz. Yogurt- & 4 oz. Pudding- Non-fat, No-added sugar	8 oz. Split Pea Soup- Low-Fat, Pain	6 oz. Chicken Noodle Soup- Low-Fat, Liquefied	6 oz. Skim Milk Mixed with ½ pack Carnation Instant Bkfst Ice, as desired	6 oz. Skim Milk Mixed with ½ pack Carnation Instant Bkfst Ice, as desired	(1) – 8 oz. Liquid Meal Replacement- Medifast	6 oz. Egg Drop Soup
Meal #4	(1) – 8 oz. Liquid Meal Replacement- Medifast	8 oz. Frozen Yogurt- Non-fat, No-added sugar	(1) – 8 oz. Liquid Meal Replacement- Medifast	(1) – 8 oz. Liquid Meal Replacement- Medifast	(1) – 8 oz. Liquid Meal Replacement- Medifast	(1) – 8 oz. Liquid Meal Replacement- Medifast	(1) – 8 oz. Liquid Meal Replacement- Medifast
Meal #5	6 oz. Tomato Soup- Prepared with Skim Milk	(1) – 8 oz. Liquid Meal Replacement- Medifast	(1) – 8 oz. Liquid Meal Replacement- Medifast	6 oz. Lentil Soup- Low-fat	6 oz. Turkey & Vegetable Soup- Low-Fat, Liquefied	6 oz. Skim Milk Mixed with ½ Scoop Alba Ice, as desired	6 oz. Skim Milk Mixed with ½ Scoop Alba Ice, as desired
Meal #6	(1) – 8 oz. Liquid Meal Replacement- Medifast	(1) – 8 oz. Liquid Meal Replacement- Medifast	(1) – 8 oz. Liquid Meal Replacement- Medifast	4 oz. Pudding– & 4 oz. Yogurt- Non-fat, No-added sugar	(1) – 8 oz. Liquid Meal Replacement- Medifast	6 oz. Fage Yogurt – Blended well with ½ cup Berries	(1) – 8 oz. Liquid Meal Replacement- Medifast

Average Calories for each day = ~ 650
Average grams of Carbohydrate each day = ~ 80

Average grams of Protein each day = ~ 70
Average grams of Fat each day = ~ 6

Week 2 - Sample Post-operative Full Liquid Menu

	Day #1	Day #2	Day #3	Day #4	Day #5	Day #6	Day #7
Meal #1	(1)– 8 oz. Liquid Meal Replacement- Medifast	(1)– 8 oz. Liquid Meal Replacement- Medifast	(1)– 8 oz. Liquid Meal Replacement- Medifast	6 oz. Skim Milk Mixed with ½ Scoop Alba Ice, as desired	(1)– 8 oz. Liquid Meal Replacement- Medifast	6 oz. Fage Yogurt– Blended well with ½ cup canned Peaches	(1)– 8 oz. Liquid Meal Replacement- Medifast
Meal #2	8 oz. Pudding– Non-fat, No-added sugar	(1)– 8 oz. Liquid Meal Replacement- Medifast	(1)– 8 oz. Liquid Meal Replacement- Medifast	(1)– 8 oz. Liquid Meal Replacement- Medifast	6 oz. Skim Milk Mixed with ½ Carnation Bkfst Ice, as desired	(1)– 8 oz. Liquid Meal Replacement- Medifast	6 oz. Skim Milk Mixed with ½ Scoop Alba Ice, as desired
Meal #3	(1)– 8 oz. Liquid Meal Replacement- Medifast	(1)– 8 oz. Liquid Meal Replacement- Medifast	6 oz. Cream of Tomato Soup- Prepared with Skim Milk	(1)– 8 oz. Liquid Meal Replacement- Medifast	(1)– 8 oz. Liquid Meal Replacement- Medifast	(1)– 8 oz. Liquid Meal Replacement- Medifast	(1)– 8 oz. Liquid Meal Replacement- Medifast
Meal #4	(1)– 8 oz. Liquid Meal Replacement- Medifast	4 oz. Yogurt– & 4 oz. Pudding- Non-fat, No-added sugar	8 oz. Pudding– Non-fat, No-added sugar	(1)– 8 oz. Liquid Meal Replacement- Medifast	8 oz. Chobani Yogurt- Non-fat, No-added sugar	(1)– 8 oz. Liquid Meal Replacement- Medifast	(1)– 8 oz. Liquid Meal Replacement- Medifast
Meal #5	6 oz. Egg Drop Soup	(1)– 8 oz. Liquid Meal Replacement- Medifast	(1)– 8 oz. Liquid Meal Replacement- Medifast	6 oz. Chicken & Rice Soup- Low-Fat, Liquefied	(1)– 8 oz. Liquid Meal Replacement- Medifast	6 oz. Split Pea Soup- Low-Fat, Plain	(1)– 8 oz. Liquid Meal Replacement- Medifast
Meal #6	(1)– 8 oz. Liquid Meal Replacement- Medifast	6 oz. Skim Milk Mixed with ½ Carnation Bkfst Ice, as desired	(1)– 8 oz. Liquid Meal Replacement- Medifast	(1)– 8 oz. Liquid Meal Replacement- Medifast	(1)– 8 oz. Liquid Meal Replacement- Medifast	(1)– 8 oz. Liquid Meal Replacement- Medifast	4 oz. Yogurt– & 4 oz. Pudding- Non-fat, No-added sugar

Average Calories for each day = ~ 650

Average grams of Carbohydrate each day = ~ 80

Average grams of Protein each day = ~ 70

Average grams of Fat each day = ~ 6

Recommended Post-Operative Nutrition Plan

MORE ON FLUIDS

Fluid, in the form of **water**, is a key component to losing weight. Although water essentially should be consumed on a near-constant basis, there are specific guidelines that will promote optimal food tolerance, as well as, help to prolong satiety while living with the Lap-Band.

These guidelines are as follows:

Reduce liquid consumption to only small sips of water beginning 15 minutes before each meal in preparation for the intake of food.

**Furthermore, and even more importantly,
it is recommended to
AVOID drinking *when eating* a meal
and in addition
AVOID drinking for *one hour following* a meal.**

If needed, you may consume small sips of water with your meal and one hour after however, the less you drink the better.

Limiting liquids to very small sips approximately fifteen minutes before the start of a meal will prevent the possibility of feeling full. A common tendency with Lap-Band treatment is to feel full after drinking a large quantity of water at a very quick pace. This occurs from water maximally distending the stomach pouch and signaling nerves of satiety. Fullness gained in this capacity is only temporary, a "pseudo fullness," which is not ideal before the beginning of a meal. When the pouch is distended from the intake of food, satiation is experienced in a more profound and long existing manner.

Limiting liquids during meals will prolong fullness through maintaining solid food consistency within the pouch. Drinking liquid at a meal (or shortly following) will inevitably soften the texture of food. When this occurs, food passes through the stomach pouch at a quicker pace, from the action of "pouch flushing." The result of this behavior is returning to hunger sooner and often a more than ideal quantity of intake. Vomiting and/or discomfort can also be experienced when a large quantity of liquid is consumed with the meal.

Limiting liquids at meals will also help to execute favorable chewing habits. In addition, a more profound satiation effect will be noted from the "feel of food" with the absence of liquid.

As a side note related to water consumption: If hunger begins to develop between meals during your solid food plan (~ 5 week), try drinking 8 to 12 ounces of water within 30 seconds. **"Water loading,"** will help achieve a temporary feeling of fullness for 20 - 30 minutes by distending the stomach pouch.

Recommended Post-Operative Nutrition Plan

Consume Soft, Mushy Foods starting at the third week following surgery.

Soft foods are generally moist and require minimal chewing before swallowing. **Use of a fork (for soft foods) or a spoon (for mushy foods) will be needed- knives will not be necessary.** Using a knife would indicate the consumption of non-advisable solid food.

Fiber must be **avoided** during this phase to help ensure optimal tolerance. This excludes all whole grain products including bread, pasta, rice, and baked potatoes. Fibrous fruits and vegetables are not advised. Salads must not be consumed during this soft, mushy phase. In addition, course meats and other tough-textured protein foods should not be consumed at this point including steak, white meat chicken and turkey, pork, veal, and shellfish.

BEHAVIOR STRATEGIES INCLUDE:

1. Consume a **soft, mushy food plan** for **two weeks-** weeks 3 and 4 post-surgery.
2. **Plan** to consume **six**, nourishing **soft, mushy meals daily.***
   ***One liquid meal replacement** is also recommended to ensure beneficial protein intake. If time is extremely limited, you may consume one or two of your six meals as a liquid meal replacement, however, make certain to consume at least four "soft, mushy" meals to help establish important intake habits such as eating slowly and learning to sense feelings of comfortable satisfaction.
3. **Space** soft, mushy **meals** approximately **2 to 3 hours apart**.
4. **Pace meals** so it takes **15 minutes** to consume a recommended **3 oz. serving**.
   Consume soft, mushy foods at a pace of approximately **1 oz. over a 5-minute period**.
5. The entire meal serving should resemble the size of a **deck of cards**.
6. Consume approximately **2 oz.** of a **protein source** and approximately **1 oz.** of a **carbohydrate source** at each meal.
7. **Protein** and **carbohydrate** foods are **listed** in **1 oz. servings**. (See pages 84 & 85)
   Since 2 ounces of protein is recommended at each meal and the portion size for each protein enriched food is labeled at a 1 oz. serving, you have the choice to either
   - choose two different protein foods consumed at a one-ounce serving (1 oz. = 2 tbsp.)
   Or
   - choose a single protein food consumed at double the serving size (2 oz = 4 tbsp.)

   ### For example:
   If tuna fish and American cheese were both desired at the same meal, then the quantity would be 2 tbsp. of tuna fish **and** one thin slice of American cheese. If either food is desired solely at the meal, then the quantity per individual item is doubled- 4 tbsp. of tuna fish **or** two thin slices of American cheese.

Recommended Post-Operative Nutrition Plan

8. **Weighing** and **measuring** are helpful techniques to determine appropriate servings. Soft foods should be weighed on the scale for appropriate measurement, whereas foods of mushy consistency can be accurately measured from tbsp. servings. If using a scale for measurement, food should always be weighed on a scale after cooking.

    Weighing and measuring food is not something that may be needed, or for that matter, is even highly recommended in the future because in weighing food, portion control is being determined by external measures (the scale) rather than internal regulation (feelings of satiety). Determining the serving of your meal based on internal regulation is what makes surgical intervention a proven success apart from conventional externally directed programs.

    The **ultimate goal** after fully adjusting to post-banded life is to determine the quantity of your meal based on internal cues. Internal cues are physical indications, which help you determine the level of intake needed to sense comfortable satisfaction. These physical indications are more profoundly recognized with the help of the Lap-Band.

9. **Stop eating when** you feel a sense of **"comfortable satisfaction."**
    Begin learning to recognize internal cues of satiation. This feeling can be described as knowing you can eat one more bite of food; however, your intuition tells you that one more bite may lead to uncomfortable fullness and the possibility for regurgitation.

10. If possible, consume the **protein source before eating** the **carbohydrate source**. Consuming protein foods first can help to both initiate and prolong satiation. In addition, your body is in need of amino acids (the building blocks of protein) to perform various enzymatic reactions including regulation of an efficient metabolism. Consuming protein at the beginning of meals will ensure adequate consumption of this key nutrient without taking space for carbohydrate based foods.

11. Although the decision is yours to make, **natural, trans-free condiments** such as butter, margarine, mayonnaise, ketchup, mustard, etc. are highly recommended. Choosing natural products are easier for your body to process, which will create better health and well-being. Adding condiments as needed to food can provide extra moisture, which may in essence help improve the ease of intake at this particular stage in your adjustment to the Band.

12. Seasonings used in cooking must be in **powdered form** (e.g., salt, pepper, onion, garlic) to allow for optimal tolerance during the soft, mushy food phase.

13. In preparation of meals, it is recommended to reduce liquid consumption to small sips of water 15 minutes before taking your first bite. *It is then further recommended to avoid drinking water when eating and for at least (at this point during the soft, mushy food plan) 30 minutes following each meal.* Since your intake consists of six meals per day with a meal every 2 - 3 hours, waiting one hour after meals will restrict the time needed for adequate water intake, thus possibly compromising hydration. Once advancing to solid foods, liquids should not be consumed for 60 minutes after each meal.

Recommended Post-Operative Nutrition Plan

Examples of (soft-mushy) protein sources include*:

* Remember to consume approximately **2 oz.** (4 tbsp.) at each of your six meals daily.

1. **Soft Cheese*** (1 oz. = 1 thin slice) (e.g., American, Muenster, and Feta) **and Cream Cheese*** (1 oz. = 2 tbsp.) *Avoid: Swiss, Mozzarella, Cheddar, and Provolone.* *If cheese is consumed regularly, try low-fat cheese for reduced calories.

2. **Soft Boiled and Poached Egg** (1 oz. = 1 egg or 2 egg whites) *Avoid: Scrambled Eggs.*

3. **Tuna Fish, Egg, Chicken, and Turkey Salad** (1 oz. = 2 tbsp.) Prepare salad with regular or lite mayo – your preference. *Avoid: Celery and Onions.*

4. **Flaked Fish** (1 oz. = 2 tbsp. cooked) (e.g., Flounder and Salmon) *Avoid: Shellfish.*

5. **Luncheon Meat** (1 oz. = 1 thin slice) (e.g., Turkey, Chicken Breast, and Ham) *Avoid: Salami, Pepperoni, Pastrami, Corn Beef, and Roast Beef*

6. **Minced, Dark Chicken & Turkey Meat with Gravy** (1 oz. = 2 tbsp. - e.g., Thigh & Leg) *Avoid White Meat Chicken and Turkey (e.g., Breast)*

7. **Grounded Beef, Chicken, and Turkey as a Meatball/Burger** (1 oz. = 2 tbsp.)

Due to less protein content, consume fewer choices daily from the following items:

8. **Soy Products** (1 oz. = 2 tbsp. - e.g., Tofu, Garden, or Veggie Burger's)

9. **Beans** (1 oz. = 2 tbsp. - all varieties of mashed beans- including mushy *Chili* as well.)

10. **Peanut Butter – Natural, Creamy, and Low-Fat** (1 oz. = 2 tbsp)

11. **Cottage Cheese*** **and Ricotta Cheese*** (1 oz. = 2 tbsp.) *Try low-fat for less calories.

12. **Soups-** low-fat, (1 oz. = ~ 1/2 cup) (All Varieties, including soups with **Chunks**.) *1 oz. serving of carbohydrate also included if soup contains rice, noodles, &/ vegetables.

Recommended Post-Operative Nutrition Plan

Examples of (soft-mushy) carbohydrate sources include*:

* Remember to consume approximately **1 oz.** (2 tbsp.) at each of your six meals daily.

1. *Crackers* (Plain, Saltine or Ritz – 5 to 6 each = one serving)

2. *Hot Cereal and Soggy Cold Cereal* (1 oz. = 2 tbsp.) *Avoid: Nuts, Dried Fruit & Clusters.* (e.g., Oatmeal, Farina, Cream of Wheat, Cheerios, Corn Flakes and Special K)

3. *Skinless, Mushy Fruit* (1 oz. = 2 tbsp.)
   (e.g., Applesauce (unsweetened), Bananas, Canned Fruit (e.g., Peaches and Pears in 100% natural juice), Berries (all varieties) (e.g., Strawberries, Blueberries, etc.) including All-Fruit Jelly, and Melons (ripe) (e.g., Honeydew, Watermelon, and Cantaloupe)
   Avoid: All fresh and canned Pineapple, Oranges, Grapefruit, along with Grapes.

4. *Well Cooked, Mushy Vegetables* (1 oz. = 2 tbsp.)
   (e.g., Creamed-Spinach, Butternut and Green Squash, Avocado, Peas, Hummus, as well as, Carrots, Cauliflower, and Turnips cooked to a mashed consistency.

5. *Mashed Potatoes* (1 oz. = 2 tbsp.—White and Sweet)
   In addition, you can consume the inside of a baked potato as long as ingredients are added to moisten the potato such as sour cream, butter, or margarine.

6. *Yogurt/Pudding/Milk/Meal Replacement Beverage such as Medifast*
   (Non-fat, No-added sugar = 6 to 8 oz. = 1 oz. serving of both protein and carbohydrate.)

7. If desired, *Baby Food* can be consumed for both your protein and carbohydrate sources.

Please Note:

It is quite common for people to require an adjustment period when transitioning their dietary intake from liquids only to soft, mushy food. This adjustment period may entail introducing one soft consistency meal daily to an already existing liquid plan. By slowly introducing one soft meal daily, intake habits are optimized while limiting the tendency for poor tolerance.

Please refer to page (87) for a transitional full liquid to soft menu. The transitional menu plan can apply as one of the two weeks recommended for the soft meal plan or just as an extra week in the overall process of adjusting to appropriate intake habits.

Recommended Post-Operative Nutrition Plan

For optimal tolerance, some patients may need to puree foods in a blender or a food processor until a semi-solid or mushy consistency is achieved.

Instructions for Pureeing Food

Preparation of Foods

1. **Meats -**   Cook ground meats in water until done. Drain, reserve cooking liquid.
2. **Poultry -**   Cut into small pieces (the size of an eraser at the end of a pencil) and cook in water until done. As an alternative, cook poultry with ¼ cup of water in microwave on medium for six to eight minutes or until done. Drain and reserve liquid.
3. **Fish Fillet -**   Steam for five to seven minutes or until opaque and flakes easily with a fork. As an alternative, cook fish in microwave with 3 tablespoons of water. Microwave on high for three to five minutes. Drain, and reserve liquid.
4. **Fruits -**   Wash and remove skin and pit/seeds, if necessary. Fruits may also be steamed lightly until tender for optimal tolerance.
5. **Vegetables -** Wash and cut into very small pieces. Steam, boil, or microwave until very tender.

Pureeing of Foods

1. Place (cooked) foods in blender or food processor.
2. Add liquid to cover meats, poultry, and/or vegetables (e.g., broth, reserve of cooking liquid, lemon juice, tomato sauce, onion soup, vegetable, or diluted fruit juice).
3. Blend until smooth like applesauce.
4. Strain out lumps and seeds.
5. Enhance flavor by experimenting with spices and herbs.

Storing Foods
Try using ice cube trays for storing pureed food portions. Each cube holds approximately 1 ounce. Freeze the food in the ice cube tray. When frozen, remove the cubes and store in a freezer bag.

Sample Optional Transitional Menu from Full Liquid to Soft, Mushy Food

	Day #1	Day #2	Day #3	Day #4	Day #5	Day #6	Day #7
Meal #1	(1)– 8 oz. Liquid Meal Replacement- Medifast	2 tbsp. Oatmeal- cooked until mushy with Skim Milk / 1 Soft Egg White	8 oz. Yogurt- Non-fat, No-added sugar	(1)– 8 oz. Liquid Meal Replacement- Medifast	(1)– 8 oz. Liquid Meal Replacement- Medifast	2 tbsp. Cream of Wheat Cereal cooked until mushy with Skim Milk / 1 Soft Egg White	1 Poached Egg / 1 sl. Muenster Cheese-Low-fat / 2 tbsp. Berries- mushy
Meal #2	(1)– 8 oz. Liquid Meal Replacement- Medifast	(1)– 8 oz. Liquid Meal Replacement- Medifast	(1)– 8 oz. Liquid Meal Replacement- Medifast	4 tbsp. Egg Salad / 1 tsp. Mayo / 6 Crackers- plain	2 sl. American Cheese- Low-fat / 5 Crackers- plain	2 tbsp. Ricotta Cheese- part-skim / 2 tbsp. Tofu- cooked to mushy / 2 tbsp. Pears- canned, 100% juice	4 tbsp. Cottage Cheese-Low-fat / 2 tbsp. Peaches- canned, 100% juice
Meal #3	4 tbsp Cottage Cheese / 2 tbsp. Peaches- canned	(1)– 8 oz. Liquid Meal Replacement- Medifast	4 tbsp. Chicken canned meat / 1 tsp. Mayo / 6 Crackers- plain	(1)– 8 oz. Liquid Meal Replacement- Medifast	1.5 cup Chicken Noodle Soup- Low-fat & Chunky	4 tbsp. Tuna Fish / 1 tsp. Mayo / 5 Crackers- plain	2 tbsp. Peanut Butter- natural, creamy, Low-fat / 2 tbsp. Banana
Meal #4	(1)– 8 oz. Liquid Meal Replacement- Medifast	4 oz. Pudding- & 4 oz. Yogurt- Non-fat, No-added sugar	(1)– 8 oz. Liquid Meal Replacement- Medifast	4 tbsp. Garden Burger- mushy / 2 tbsp. Carrots- cooked until mushy	(1)– 8 oz. Liquid Meal Replacement- Medifast	(1)– 8 oz. Liquid Meal Replacement- Medifast	4 tbsp. Chili / Grated Cheese / 6 Crackers- plain
Meal #5	6 oz. Skim Milk Mixed with ½ scoop Alba Ice, as desired	(1)– 8 oz. Liquid Meal Replacement- Medifast	2 oz. Meatball Sauce to taste / 2 tbsp. Creamed Spinach	2 oz. Swordfish- baked / 2 tbsp. Sweet Potato- mushy	2 oz. Turkey- grounded, burger patty / 2 tbsp. Yellow Squash- mushy	2 oz. Chicken minced, dark meat with gravy / 2 tbsp. Mashed Potato	2 oz. Fish Fillet- grilled / 2 tbsp. Peas- mushy
Meal #6	(1)– 8 oz. Liquid Meal Replacement- Medifast	2 sl. Muenster Cheese-Low-fat / 5 Crackers- plain	8 oz. Pudding- Non-fat, No-added sugar	4 oz. Yogurt- & 4 oz. Pudding- Non-fat, No-added sugar	2 tbsp. Peanut Butter- natural, creamy, low-fat / 1 tbsp. Jelly- All fruit / 6 Crackers- plain	1.5 cup Turkey & Vegetable Soup Low-fat & Chunky	(1)– 8 oz. Liquid Meal Replacement- Medifast

Average Calories for each day = ~ 700
Average grams of Carbohydrate each day = ~ 85

Average grams of Protein each day = ~ 75
Average grams of Fat each day = ~ 8

Week 3 - Sample Soft, Mushy Food Menu: Nutrient value also includes one liquid meal replacement beverage daily

	Day #1	Day #2	Day #3	Day #4	Day #5	Day #6	Day #7
Meal #1	4 Tbsp Cottage Cheese- Low-fat. Pears- canned, 100% juice	1 Poached Egg 1 sl. American Cheese- Low-fat 2 tbsp. Strawberries- mushy	2 tbsp. Peanut Butter- natural, creamy, Low-fat 2 tbsp. Banana	2 Soft Boiled Egg Whites 2 tbsp. Cream of Wheat cooked until mushy with Skim Milk	2 sl. American Cheese- Low-fat 2 tbsp. Cheerios- mushy 2 oz. Skim Milk	1 Poached Egg 1 sl. Muenster Cheese- Low-fat 2 tbsp. Farina- cooked until mushy with Skim Milk	4 tbsp. Cottage Cheese- Low-fat 2 Tbsp Peaches- canned, 100% juice
Meal #2	1 sl. American Cheese- Low-fat 2 tbsp. Oatmeal cooked until mushy with Skim Milk	4 tbsp. Tuna Fish 1 oz. Avocado	2 tbsp. Kidney Beans- mashed 1 oz. Feta Cheese- Low-fat 2 tbsp. Sweet Potato- mashed	2 oz. Tofu- cooked until mushy 2 tbsp. Yellow Squash-cooked to mushy, mixed & flavored with Tofu	2 oz. Feta Cheese- Low-fat 1 tbsp. Hummus 1 tbsp. Creamed Spinach	2 tbsp. Peanut Butter- natural, creamy, Low-fat 2 tbsp. Jelly- All Fruit 6 Crackers- plain	2 sl. Chicken- luncheon meat, sliced thin 2 tbsp. Applesauce- unsweetened
Meal #3	1.5 cup Chicken Vegetable Soup- Low-fat & Chunky	2 sl. Turkey- luncheon meat, sliced thin 2 tbsp. Carrots- cooked until mushy	1 cup All Beef Soup- Low-fat & Chunky 2 tbsp. Creamed Spinach	4 tbsp. Cottage Cheese- Low-fat 2 tbsp. Blackberries- mushy	6 oz. Yogurt- Non-fat, No-added sugar 2 tbsp. Raspberries- mushy	1 cup Lentil Soup 2 tbsp. (ripe) Honeydew Melon	4 tbsp. Tofu- cooked to mushy 2 tbsp. Cauliflower- cooked to mushy, mixed & flavored with Tofu
Meal #4	4 tbsp. Turkey- canned meat 1 tsp. Mayo 2 tbsp. Mashed Potato	1 cup Split Pea Soup- Low-fat 6 Crackers-plain	2 sl Ham- Low-fat luncheon meat, sliced thin 2 tbsp. Applesauce- unsweetened	4 tbsp. Chili- mushy 1 oz. Parmesan Grated Cheese 6 Crackers- plain	4 tbsp. Chicken canned meat 1 tsp. Mayo 6 Crackers-plain	2 oz. Garden Burger- mushy 2 tbsp. Creamed Spinach- mushy	4 tbsp. Egg Salad 1 tsp. Mayo 6 Crackers- plain
Meal #5	2 oz. Fish Fillet- grilled 2 tbsp. Creamed Spinach	2 oz. Chicken- minced, dark meat with gravy 2 tbsp. Green Squash- cooked until mushy	2 oz. Garden Burger- mushy 2 tbsp. Peas- cooked until mushy	2 oz. Salmon- broiled 2 tbsp. Cauliflower- cooked until mushy	2 oz. Meatball mushy Sauce to taste 2 tbsp. Carrots cooked until mushy	2 oz. Turkey- minced, dark meat with gravy 2 tbsp. Sweet Potato- mashed	2 oz. Hamburger Patty- mushy 2 tbsp. Mashed Potato
Meal #6	2 sl. Muenster Cheese- Low-fat 1 oz. Avocado	8 oz. Yogurt- Non-fat, No-added sugar	8 oz. Pudding Non-fat, No-added sugar	1.5 cup Turkey & Rice Soup- Low-fat & Chunky	4 tbsp. Ricotta Cheese- Low-fat 2 tbsp. Jelly- All Fruit	8 oz. Pudding Non-fat, No-added sugar	8 oz. Yogurt Non-fat, No-added sugar

Average Total Calories each day = ~ 800
Average Total Grams of Carbohydrate each day = ~ 90

Average Total Grams of Protein each day = ~ 80
Average Total Grams of Fat each day = ~ 15

Week 4 - Sample Soft, Mushy Food Menu: Nutrient value also includes one liquid meal replacement beverage daily

	Day #1	Day #2	Day #3	Day #4	Day #5	Day #6	Day #7
Meal #1	2 Soft Boiled Egg Whites 2 tbsp. Farina- cooked until mushy with Skim Milk	1 sl. American Cheese- Low-fat 2 tbsp. Special K Cereal- mushy 2 oz. Skim Milk	2 Poached Egg Whites 2 tbsp. Oatmeal- cooked until mushy with Skim Milk	6 oz. Yogurt- Non-fat, No-added sugar 2 tbsp. Blackberries- mushy	2 sl. Muenster Cheese- Low-fat 2 tbsp. Farina- cooked until mushy with Skim Milk	1 Poached Egg 1 sl. American Cheese- Low-fat 2 tbsp. Blueberries- mushy	1 tbsp. Cream Cheese- plain 1 tbsp. Peanut Butter- natural, creamy, Low-fat 6 Crackers-plain
Meal #2	2 oz. Feta Cheese- Low-fat 2 tbsp. Hummus	4 tbsp. Cottage Cheese- Low-fat 2 tbsp. Peaches- canned, 100% juice	2 sl Ham- Low-fat 2 tbsp. Applesauce- unsweetened	2 sl. Chicken- Luncheon meat, sliced thin 1 oz. Avocado	2 tbsp. Peanut Butter- natural, creamy, Low-fat 2 tbsp. Banana	1.5 cup Cream of Broccoli Soup- Low-fat & Chunky	2 Soft Boiled Egg Whites 2 tbsp. Farina- cooked to mushy with Skim Milk
Meal #3	2 tbsp. Chili- mushy 1 oz. Parmesan Grated Cheese 2 tbsp. Peas- mushy	2 oz. Garden Burger- mushy 2 tbsp. Carrots- cooked until mushy	4 tbsp. Egg Salad 1 tsp. Mayo 5 Crackers- plain	1 sl. Muenster Cheese- Low-fat ½ cup Cream of Chicken Soup- Low-fat & Chunky 5 Crackers -plain	2 tbsp. Kidney Beans- mashed 1 oz. Parmesan Grated Cheese 2 tbsp. Mashed Potato	2 oz. Chicken- gravy minced, dark meat 2 tbsp. Sweet Potato- mushy	2 oz. Tofu- cooked to mushy 2 tbsp. Yellow Squash-cooked to mushy, mixed & flavored with Tofu
Meal #4	2 sl. Turkey- luncheon meat, sliced thin 2 tbsp. (ripe) Watermelon	1 cup Egg Drop Soup with One Wonton Noodle 6 Crackers- plain	4 tbsp. Ricotta Cheese-part- skim 2 tbsp. Jelly- All Fruit	2 oz Garden Burger- mushy 2 tbsp. Carrots- cooked until mushy	2 sl. Chicken- luncheon meat, sliced thin 2 tbsp. Peaches- canned, 100% juice	2 sl. Ham -Low-fat luncheon meat, sliced thin 2 tbsp. Pears- canned, 100% juice	8 oz. Pudding Non-fat, No- added sugar
Meal #5	2 oz. Flounder- broiled 2 tbsp. Creamed Spinach	2 oz. Meatball- mushy Sauce to taste 2 tbsp. Cauliflower- mushy	1.5 cup Chicken Noodle Soup- Low-fat & Chunky	2 oz. Tofu- cooked until mushy 2 tbsp. Yellow Squash- cooked to mushy, mixed & flavored with Tofu	2 oz. Halibut- grilled 2 tbsp. Butternut Squash-mushy	2 oz. Vegetable Burger- mushy 2 tbsp. Turnips- mushy	2 oz. Turkey grounded, burger patty 2 tbsp. Avocado
Meal #6	2 tbsp. Peanut Butter- natural, creamy, Low-fat 2 tbsp. Banana	4 oz. Pudding & 4 oz. Yogurt- Non-fat. No- added sugar	4 Tbsp Tuna Fish 1 tsp. Mayo 6 Crackers- plain	8 oz. Pudding Non-fat, No-added sugar	6 oz. Yogurt- Non-fat, No- added sugar 2 tbsp. (ripe) Honeydew Melon	2 sl. Muenster Cheese- Low-fat 2 tbsp. Applesauce- unsweetened	1.5 cup Turkey Vegetable Soup- Low-fat & Chunky

Average Total Calories each day = ~ 800
Average Total Grams of Carbohydrate each day = ~ 90

Average Total Grams of Protein each day = ~ 80
Average Total Grams of Fat each day = ~ 15

Recommended Post-Operative Nutrition Plan

With successful completion of a soft, mushy food plan, you are now ready to begin consuming solid food. *Keep in mind; if you have not "mastered" the habit of eating slowly,* you should still consider consuming soft foods for a longer duration because all solid food must be thoroughly chewed before swallowing to promote optimal tolerance.

Consume Solid Foods starting at the fifth week after surgery.

Behavior Strategies Include:

1. **Plan** to consume **3**, nourishing **solid meals daily, along** with an **optional 4ᵗʰ mini-meal**. Consuming 6 meals a day at this point in time may diminish the effective use of surgery because optimal satiation of intake may not occur while eating multiple, small meals.

   BREAKFAST IS KEY – Have your first meal within 2 hours upon awakening. Waiting to eat until late in the day increases a tendency for poor tolerance of food. Additionally, the body requires food for proper metabolic functioning. By not eating, your metabolism slows down and the body holds onto stored fat as a protective measure.
2. **Space** solid **meals** approximately **5 hours apart** to help avoid the tendency to snack.
3. **Cut food** with a **knife** into **bite size** portion **before** beginning your **meal**.
4. **Pace** solid **meals** so it takes **20 minutes** to consume. Taking less time means the meal has been consumed too quickly and probably not chewed well. It may also indicate that in fact not enough food was consumed at the meal. Taking longer at a meal (45 - 60 minutes) usually leads to over consumption and additional calories.
5. **Chew** all **food** to a **"mushy" consistency.** Chew solid food until the texture is mushy in your mouth before swallowing to reduce the possibility of gastrointestinal complications.
6. In preparation for your meal, it is recommended to reduce the consumption of liquids to small sips of water 15 minutes before the start of the meal. It is further recommended to **avoid drinking when eating** and for **60 minutes following** each **meal**.
7. **Choose quality food** to help **promote** a **prolonged** feeling of **fullness**.

AN OPTIMAL MEAL CONSISTS OF:
LEAN PROTEIN – FINELY CUT-UP
(I.E., CHICKEN, TURKEY, BEEF, FISH)
WITH RAW, GRILLED OR STEAMED VEGETABLES.

As a general guideline, **3 ounces of protein** and **2 ounces of vegetables** are recommended at each meal. **Portion size** is dependent upon many individual factors, which are discussed in detail in other sections of your education material.

Recommended Post-Operative Nutrition Plan

Although meals will vary in content, a combination of protein-based foods and vegetables will assist in helping to achieve complete satiation. This sense of satiation will extend for a prolonged period to promote hours of satiety, which is fundamental to the effective use of your surgical tool and ultimately obtaining a healthy weight.

It is best to, **consume protein-based foods and vegetables first at meals** followed by the intake of a carbohydrate-based food. If you decide to omit eating a vegetable, it is then recommended to increase the quantity of your protein (food) rather than consuming a larger serving of a carbohydrate (food).

You may choose to balance your optimal meal of lean protein and vegetable
in the months ahead with…

One of the following Carbohydrate Choices:

1. ***Bread*-** Recommended portion size is 1 slice.
   Bread products tend to be very difficult to tolerate because of the expansion of dough, which causes a "sponge-like" effect within the stomach pouch. Therefore, they are not generally recommended for regular consumption. Doughy breads in particular, such as bagels, rolls, and Italian bread are especially challenging to tolerate. Bread products that contain less dough are significantly easier to tolerate. These breads include: *reduced calorie bread (40 calorie per slice), pita, wraps, and flat breads.*
   In addition, ***TOASTING*** bread products has helped to improve tolerance.

2. ***Pasta, Rice, and Healthy Whole Grains*** (e.g., Millet, Quinoa, Spelt, Buckwheat)
   All Pasta, **Rice, and Whole Grains products** must be consumed with extreme **caution** because these items tend to expand and swell once consumed and may lead to discomfort and poor tolerance. Pay careful attention to the portion size you are consuming. It is recommended to begin with an intake of **only 1 - 2 ounces (2- 4 tbsp.) cooked** and then proceed to a larger intake depending on the degree of tolerance. Experimentation with different varieties of pasta, rice, and whole grains may be needed to determine the type that will provide for consistent, optimal tolerance.

3. ***Potato*** (**baked or boiled, skin is tolerated** when chewed to a mushy consistency)
   Recommended portion size is 3 ounces.

4. ***Fruit*** (**fresh, skin is tolerated** when chewed to a mushy consistency)
   Recommended portion size is 1 small size fresh fruit, ½ medium size fresh fruit, or ½ cup canned fruit (preferably unsweetened).

5. ***Cereal*** (**all varieties,** preferably unsweetened)
   Recommended portion size is ½ cup.

Recommended Post-Operative Nutrition Plan

Keep in Mind:

Bread, Pasta, Rice, Red Meat (e.g., steak and pork), Shellfish,
and
Fibrous Fruits and Vegetables (e.g., celery, asparagus, and pineapple)

Maybe difficult to tolerate and can cause discomfort and/or vomiting.

It is important to recognize that these foods fill up the pouch quickly even when you take bite size portions. Introduce each food separately and if you cannot tolerate a food, then it is advised to **WAIT ONE MONTH BEFORE TRYING THAT FOOD AGAIN.**

By waiting a month or longer to reintroduce foods that were poorly tolerated, improvement of habits can more easily occur as time is provided to do so. In addition, some level of anxiety may have developed because of regurgitating and/or vomiting. Briefly dissociating from the intake of that particular food may make it easier to reintroduce this food at a later time.

TIPS:

Regurgitation, pain, and discomfort are common if you eat…
Tough, Chewy, and/or Dry Meat.

Try **marinades** (along with lemon, orange juice, and salt), slicing finely (shaving), or cooking slowly in a **casserole** or **crock-pot** to tenderize meats well. Also, instead of cooking at 350° degrees for 40 minutes, seal the top of the pan in foil (tight seal) and cook for 60 to 120 minutes at 275° to 300° degrees.

Some banded individuals have noted that the order in which they eat foods can make a difference with tolerance. If there is a food that is difficult to tolerate, it may be of benefit for a short period to consume foods of softer consistency at the beginning of the meal followed by foods that are solid and digest more slowly.

For example, You may decide to consume your meal in the following order to allow for improved tolerance: Soup, Mashed Potato, Vegetable, and Meat*.

*Once meat and vegetables are well tolerated, it is always best to eat these foods first at the meal to obtain quicker and more profound satiation.

It is quite common for people to require an adjustment period when transitioning their dietary intake from soft, mushy food to solid consistency. This adjustment period may entail introducing one solid consistency meal daily to an already existing soft, mushy food plan. By slowly introducing one solid meal daily, intake habits are optimized while limiting the tendency for poor tolerance. Please refer to page (95) for a transitional soft to solid food menu.

Sample Optional Transitional Menu from Soft Food to Solid Food

	Day #1	Day #2	Day #3	Day #4	Day #5	Day #6	Day #7
Meal #1	1 Hard Boiled Egg, 4 oz. Oatmeal, 2 oz. Skim Milk	1 Bkfst Sausage- Morning Star, 4 oz. Farina, 2 oz. Skim Milk	1 Scrambled Egg, 4 oz. Cold Cereal- with clusters, 6 oz. Skim Milk	1 sl. Swiss Cheese- Low-fat, 4 oz. Cold Cereal- with clusters, 6 oz. Skim Milk	4 oz. Cottage- Cheese- Low-fat, 3 oz. Pineapple- canned, crushed	1 Sunnyside Cooked Egg, 6 oz. Cold Cereal- with clusters, 8 oz. Skim Milk	1 Bkfst Sausage- Morning Star, 3 oz. Oatmeal, 3 oz. Blueberries
Meal #2	Nothing	10 oz. Skim Milk, 1 Banana- (blended)	1 oz. Peanut Butter- chunky ok, 1 oz. Cream Cheese- Low-fat, 6 Pretzels- Whole Wheat	Nothing	½ Meal Replacement Bar- Pure Protein, Zone, Luna, or Medifast	Nothing	Nothing
Meal #3	1 sl. Swiss Cheese- Low-fat, 1 sl. Turkey Breast, 1 Wrap- (small, toasted), Mustard- to taste, 8 Grapes	2 sl. Turkey Pastrami, 2 sl. Whole Wheat Bread (40 calorie per slice, toasted), 1 Apple- small	4 oz. Tuna Fish Small Salad- Shredded lettuce, 2 oz. Orange Sl. Dressing- Low-fat, 3 Breadsticks	3 oz. Turkey Burger, 3 oz. Baked Potato- butter, 1 Peach- small	2 sl. Chicken Breast- 2 sl. Whole Wheat Bread (40 calorie per slice, toasted), Mustard - to taste, 1 Pear- small	3 oz. Buffalo Burger, 10 Sweet Potato Fries- organic, 4 oz. Melon- cut	2 sl. Ham, 2 sl. Whole Wheat Bread (40 calorie per slice, toasted), Mustard- to taste, 4 oz. Grapefruit
Meal #4	1 cup Chunky Chicken & Vegetable Soup, 3 Breadsticks	4 oz. Chunky Chili, 6 Crackers- Whole Wheat	Nothing	2 sl. American Cheese- Low-fat, 2 sl. Whole Wheat Bread- (40 calorie, grilled) mustard	Nothing	1 oz. Peanut Butter- natural, Low-fat, chunky ok, 3 oz. Banana	Nothing
Meal #5	3 oz. Chicken Breast Gravy- to Taste, 2 oz. Squash, 2 oz. Sweet Potato- Skin ok	3 oz. Meatloaf Gravy- to taste, 2 oz. String Beans- steamed, 2 oz. Baked Potato	3 oz. Swordfish, 2 oz. Turnip Greens- mushy, 1 oz. (cooked) Rice- any type	3 oz. Meatball, 1 oz. Ricotta Ch, 1 oz. Peas, 1 oz. (cooked) Pasta- any type	2 oz. Veal, 3 oz. Broccoli- steamed, 1 oz. (cooked) Couscous	3 oz. Riblets Sauce- to taste, 3 oz. Cauliflower- steamed, 1 oz. – (cooked) Millet Grains	2 oz. Pork Small Salad- Shredded lettuce Dressing- Low-fat, 1 oz. (cooked) Quinoa Grains
Meal #6	8 oz. Yogurt- Non-fat, No-added sugar, 2 oz. Nuts	Nothing	8 oz. Pudding- Non-fat, No-added sugar, 3 oz. Banana	3 oz. Butternut Squash, 2 Breadsticks	8 oz. Yogurt- Non-fat, No-added sugar, 2 oz. Nuts	Nothing	2 oz. Cream Cheese, 6 crackers- Whole Wheat

Average Total Calories each day = each day ~ 900
Average Total Grams of Carbohydrate each day = ~ 100

Average Total Grams of Protein each day = ~ 85
Average Total Grams of Fat each day = ~ 18

Week 5 and Beyond- Sample Solid Menu

	Day #1	Day #2	Day #3	Day #4	Day #5	Day #6	Day #7
Meal #1	2 sl. String Cheese- Low-fat 6 Whole Wheat Crackers 4 oz. Mixed Fruit- cut-up	1 Egg-scrambled 1 sl. Swiss Cheese- Low-fat 1 sl. Whole Wheat Bread- (40 calorie, toasted) 1 Peach- small	2 tbsp. Cream Cheese- Low-fat 1 tbsp. Jelly- All Fruit 4 oz. Whole Grain Muffin (toasted)	1 tbsp. Peanut Butter- natural, low-fat, chunky 6- Whole Wheat Crackers 1 tbsp. Jelly- All Fruit	6 oz. Oatmeal 3 oz. Skim Milk 2 oz. Raisin- mixed in cereal with milk	1 Sunnyside Egg 1 Bkfst Sausage- Morning Star 1 sl. Whole Grain Bread- (40 calorie, toasted)	1 sl. Mozzarella Cheese- Low-fat 6 oz. Farina 3 oz. Skim Milk
Meal #2	3 oz. Chicken Breast- roasted 1 cup Salad- Shredded lettuce 1 tbsp. Dressing- Low-fat 3 oz. Fresh Orange Slices- cut-up in salad	3 oz. Garden Burger 1 Pita- (small, toasted) 10 Grapes	4 oz. Tuna 1 tbsp. Mayo 2 sl. Whole Wheat Bread (40 calorie per slice, toasted) ½ Apple	3 sl. Turkey Breast- luncheon meat ½ Tortilla Wrap (toasted)- mustard 3 oz. Pineapple	4 oz. Chicken- canned meat 1 tbsp. Mayo 1 Pita- (small, toasted) 1 Plum- small	1 Grilled Cheese Sandwich made from 2 sl. American Cheese- Low-fat 2 sl. Whole Wheat Bread- (40 calorie, grilled)- mustard	3 oz. Turkey Burger 1 cup Salad- shredded lettuce 1 tbsp. Dressing- Low-fat 3 oz. Pear- cut-up in salad
Meal #3	3 oz. Shellfish- any type 3 oz. Green Squash- steamed 3 oz. Baked Potato- skin ok 1 tbsp. Sour Cream- Low-fat	3 oz. Lean Beef- broiled 4 oz. Carrots- steamed 2 oz. (cooked) Spinach Noodles	3 oz. Veal- broiled 4 oz. Acorn Squash 6 oz. Salad- Shredded lettuce 1 tbsp. Dressing- Low-fat	4 oz. Swordfish- grilled 3 oz. Spinach- steamed 2 oz. (cooked) Spelt Grains	3 oz. Meatball 3 oz. Cauliflower- steamed 2 oz. (cooked) Whole Wheat Pasta with Sauce	3 oz. Salmon- baked 3 oz. Broccoli- steamed 3 oz. Sweet Potato- skin ok	2 oz. Pork Chop- broiled 3 oz. String Beans- steamed 2 oz. (cooked) Kamut Grains
Meal #4	2 Graham Crackers 1 tbsp. Cream Cheese- Low-fat	½ Meal Replacement Bar- Zone, Luna, Pure Protein or Medifast	4 oz. Frozen Berries with 2 tbsp. Whipped Cream- light	8 oz. Frozen Yogurt- Non-fat, No-added sugar 1 tbsp. Nuts	½ Meal Replacement Bar- Zone, Luna, Pure Protein or Medifast	2 tbsp. Cream Cheese 2 oz. Whole Wheat Pretzell	8 oz. Yogurt- Non-fat, No-added sugar 4 oz. Fruit- cut-up

Average Calories each day = ~ 1000
Average grams of Carbohydrate each day = ~ 115

Average grams of Protein each day = ~ 85
Average grams of Fat each day = ~ 22

Recommended Post-Operative Nutrition Plan

Possessing an expertise in nutrition is not such a crucial component in living with the Lap-Band. It can be very empowering however to learn a few basics about healthful eating.

Choosing a healthy diet requires familiarity with macronutrients: Protein, Carbohydrate, and Fat.

The following is a general guideline for bariatric recipients. Guidelines are dependent upon gender, age, weight, exercise and activity participation and medical history.

Early post-operative period = first month.

Calories = ~ 500 to 800 with a minimum of 70 grams of protein each day.

Rapid weight loss period = two to six months.

Calories = ~ 800 to 1000 with a range of 75 to 85 grams of protein each day.

Progressive weight loss period = six to twelve months.

Calories = ~ 1000 to 1200 with a range of 85 to 90 grams of protein each day.

Beyond twelve months =

Estimated needs are more importantly dependent upon weight loss success and activity level.

A general daily guideline beyond one-year post-surgery =

Calories = 1200 to 1400
Protein = 30 percent of calories (90 to 105 grams)
Carbohydrate = 45 percent of calories (135 to 160 grams)
Fat = 25 percent (35 to 40 grams)

Recommended Post-Operative Nutrition Plan

A simple guideline to help obtain your protein, carbohydrate & fat needs:

Seven grams of **protein** can be obtained from the following foods:

(1) ounce, cooked:	lean beef
	chicken
	turkey
	fish
(1) slice:	luncheon meat
	cheese
(2) tbsp.:	tuna fish
(1):	whole egg
(2):	egg whites
(¼) cup:	egg substitutes
(8) ounces:	milk
	yogurt
(¼) cup:	cottage cheese/ricotta cheese
(4) ounces:	tofu, tempeh
(½) cup:	beans/chickpeas
(2) tbsp.:	peanut butter

Fifteen grams of **carbohydrates** can be obtained from the following foods:

(1) slice or (1 oz.):	bread
(1) small:	fresh fruit
(½) cup:	canned fruit (unsweetened)
(1 ½) cups:	vegetables- raw, cooked, frozen, canned-all types other than peas and corn
(½) cup:	peas and corn
(½) cup, cooked:	pasta
	rice
	mashed potato
	whole grains, (e.g., millet, quinoa, spelt, buckwheat)
(3) oz:	baked potato
(½) cup:	cooked cereal
(¾) cup:	dry cereal (unsweetened)

Recommended Post-Operative Nutrition Plan

Five grams of **fat** can be obtained from the following foods:

(1) tsp.:	oil, butter, margarine, dressing
(1) tbsp.:	of all reduced calorie items

Recommended Post-Operative Nutrition Plan

MAKING THE MOST OF YOUR DAILY INTAKE:

A. **STOP EATING AT THE FIRST SIGN OF FEELING COMFORTABLY SATISFIED WITH THE QUANTITY OF FOOD CONSUMED.**
Using the physical limitation imposed by overfilling the pouch to end a meal indicates that adaptation to internal cues is not the primary guiding force to reducing your intake. Eating based on internal regulation is not the primary guiding force to reducing intake. Eating based on internal regulation is the key to successfully utilizing your surgical tool to meet your physical, nutritional, and emotional needs. Eating to a level of "comfortable satiation" will also ensure long-term maintenance of the structural integrity of your stomach pouch. Feeling uncomfortably full after a meal is an indication of eating too much at one time and can lead to eventually stretching the pouch.

Limit all distractions (e.g., eating in front of the TV, on the go, in the car, reading while eating) when consuming food to help you consciously connect with the body-mind association of your pouch and brain. Eating while in a relaxed and non-distracted environment will also ensure that you eat slowly and chew food to a proper mushy consistency before swallowing.

Most patients will experience an overfilled feeling of intake from time to time; however, it should not become a continuous pattern. The goal is to learn from any experience of uncomfortable intake, so that it does not become a chronic problem. If you overeat, the stomach pouch will be irritated for up to twelve hours. While the pouch is irritated, food tolerance will be limited with even small amounts of food causing the overfilled feeling to recur. Allow the stomach pouch to recover by **consuming only liquids for the meal at hand followed by soft, mushy foods for the next meal.**

B. **EAT ADEQUATE PROTEIN AT EACH MEAL.**
Consume a minimum of 3 ounces of lean protein at each meal. Protein-rich foods distend the pouch and help achieve and sustain adequate satiation. Additionally, your quantity of food is limited; therefore, it is important to consume foods that supply your body with high quality amino acids. Foods rich in protein include meat, chicken, turkey, fish, cheese, eggs, soy products, and beans.

C. **DRINK LIQUIDS BETWEEN MEALS (not with or shortly after a meal).**
By limiting your fluids fifteen minutes before and sixty minutes after meals, food will stay in your pouch longer and help prolong fullness.

Recommended Post-Operative Nutrition Plan

FAVORABLE HABITS	HABITS THAT ARE NOT AS FAVORABLE
1. Eat food for meals.	Drink liquid for meals.
2. Plan three meals, evenly spaced.	Lack of planning leads to skipping meals or grazing.
3. Consume protein foods first at meal then, non-starchy vegetables with starchy carbohydrates and fruits last.	Consume all carbohydrate-type food first at meal with protein foods last.
4. Eat at meals, drink liquids between meals.	Drinking when eating and during the hour after each meal
5. Eat slowly ~ twenty minutes/meal while chewing food to mushy.	Eating a meal over thirty minutes without chewing food to mushy
6. Cut all food into eraser size pieces and consume one piece per bite, place utensils down between each bite of food.	Eating chunks of food at each bite Food should be in the hand or the mouth, but not both at the same time.
7. Utilize baby spoons, cocktail forks, and smaller plates.	Utilizing normal size utensils and serving plates.
8. Measure food to learn appropriate portion sizes.	Avoid on-going measurements, however re-evaluating every three months helps stay on track.
9. Add seasoning, as desired.	Eating foods poor in flavor.
10. Stand or take a leisurely walk after a meal.	Reclining after meal or eating close to bedtime.

Bibliography

Allergan - Lap-Band System, 2011.

Allred, J.B. "Too Much of a Good Thing? An Overemphasis on Eating Low-fat Foods May be Contributing to the Alarming Increase in Overweight Among U.S. Adults." *Journal of the American Dietetic Association 95 (1995): 417-418.*

Buchwald, H. "Evolution of Operative Procedures for the Management of Morbid Obesity 1950-2000." *Obesity Surgery* 12 (2002): 705-717.

Buchwald, H. "Bariatric Surgery for Morbid Obesity: Health Implications for Patients, Health Professionals, and Third-party Payers." *Surgery for Obesity and Related Diseases* 200 (2005): 593-604.

Buffington, C. "Obesity Research." *Beyond Change* 12 (2004): 1-3.

Craig, M.R., A.R. Kristal, C.L. Cheney, and A.L. Shattuck. "The Prevalence and Impact of 'Atypical' Days in 4-day Food Records." *Journal of the American Dietetic Association* 100 (2000): 421-422.

Deitel, M. "Overweight and Obesity Worldwide Now Estimated to Involve 1.7 Billion People." *Obesity Surgery* 13: (2003) 329-330.

Dixon, J.B. "Research Update and Opportunities III." *Surgery for Obesity and Related Diseases* 1 (2005): 348-352.

Favretti, F., G. Enźi, and E. Pizzirani. "Adjustable Silicone Gastric Banding (ASGB): The Italian Experience." *Obesity Surgery* 3 (1993): 53-56.

Martin, L.F., *Obesity Research, The Severity of the Obesity Epidemic,* Ed. 1, The McGraw-Hill Co., Inc. (2004) p. 22-25, 33, 57.

United Health Organization *Obesity: Preventing and Managing the Global Epidemic* (Technical report series No. 894). Geneva: WHO, 2000.

www.ingramcontent.com/pod-product-compliance
Lightning Source LLC
Chambersburg PA
CBHW081137170526
45165CB00008B/2712